Contemporary 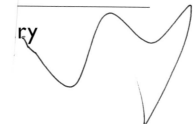 **ry**
Care Nursing

Contemporary Issues in Coronary Care Nursing

Fiona Timmins

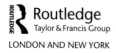

Routledge
Taylor & Francis Group

LONDON AND NEW YORK

First published 2005
by Routledge
2 Park Square, Milton Park, Abingdon, Oxon OX14 4RN

Simultaneously published in the USA and Canada by Routledge
270 Madison Ave, New York, NY 10016

Routledge is an imprint of the Taylor & Francis Group

© 2005 Fiona Timmins

Typeset in 10/12 Sabon by Wearset Ltd, Boldon, Tyne and Wear
Printed and bound in Great Britain by TJ International, Padstow, Cornwall

British Library Cataloguing in Publication Data
A catalogue record for this book is available from the British Library

Library of Congress Cataloging in Publication Data
A catalog record for this book has been requested

ISBN 0–415–30971–9 (hbk)
ISBN 0–415–30972–7 (pbk)

'Like many fathers, he had a favorite ritual: to put his whole family in the car and drive. It didn't matter where, what mattered was that he was at the wheel.'

Signe Hammer (c.1946) American author

Thanks dad for being at the wheel when I needed you . . .

Contents

Acknowledgements

The support and encouragement of many people contributed to the development and completion of this book. I would like to especially thank Sr Kay Murphy, Coronary Care, St James's Hospital Dublin, for her early and continued support. I would also like to acknowledge the early guidance of Mrs Breda Reville, Nurse Tutor, St James's Hospital Dublin. The services and facilities of Trinity College Dublin were crucial aspects of successful completion, in particular the library services and staff at the John Stearne Library, with special thanks to Virginia. I was also fortunate to be granted sabbatical leave by the college to complete the book for which I am extremely grateful.

I would like to thank those from whom I received assistance with chapter development – Sr Kay Murphy, Coronary Care, St James's Hospital Dublin; Nathalie Pallen, Staff Nurse, St James's Hospital Dublin; Michele Hughes, Lecturer University College Cork and the staff at the Coronary Care Unit, University Hospital Cork.

I cannot forget Eimear Ging who typed and retyped . . . thank you.

I would also like to thank my family, Ben, Kerry-Anne and Nathan, for making everything so worthwhile.

Foreword

Cardiac care, and especially coronary care and the role of nurses and nursing within it, has changed markedly over the past decade. The evidence-base has improved substantially and the organisation and delivery of services have changed radically. Even the diagnostic labels applied to patients have changed, with the emergence of acute coronary syndromes. Prevention and rehabilitation have, somewhat belatedly, assumed increasing importance. Nurses continue to play a pivotal role but this is ever changing in order to keep up with the advances in medicine, science and technology, emergence of new knowledge, an ageing population and the increased expectations of patients and their families as well as of nurses and other health professionals.

This book, which emphasises the nursing role in coronary care, is a welcome addition to the literature, complementing the growing number of other books on cardiac and coronary care available on the market. It is very much focused on the perspective of the nurse and nursing, with coverage of nursing theory, care planning, risk factor management, patient education, research utilisation and nurse-led services. It is clear when reading the book that it is written by an enthusiastic and committed cardiac nurse.

Its primary target audience is students and nurses working in coronary care. I am sure they will find it an invaluable resource.

Professor David R. Thompson BSc MA PhD MBA RN FRCN FESC
May 2004

Chapter 1

Nursing theory in coronary care

Key points
• The utilisation of nursing theory and conceptual models of nursing is necessary for the advancement of nursing. • The implementation of conceptual-model-based practice requires a rigorous, systematic and collegial approach. • The selection of a conceptual model for practice is dependent upon the beliefs and values held by the organisation or department. • Critical appraisal of conceptual models is an essential component of the utilisation process.

Introduction to nursing theory

> Nurses are responsible for the care they provide for their patient. They have to be active, competent and autonomous in providing this care and be able to justify what they do. It is no longer acceptable for nurses to base care on ritual and tradition – they must be able to justify the decisions they have made about appropriate care and treatment on the basis of professional expertise.
>
> (McSherry et al. 2002: 1)

Stewart (2002) suggested that cardiac nursing is 'at a crossroads of an important moment in its history'. Having abandoned what he terms 'archaic' rituals such as confining patients to bed following myocardial infarction, he suggests that nursing 'can be proud of its efforts to create new ways of caring for patients'. However, the extent to which nursing has abandoned these rituals and adopted new practices is unclear.

This notion of ritualistic or task-oriented care, although perceived as predominantly a feature of the past, is a potential feature of new nursing roles. The expanding cardiovascular nurse roles (Riley et al. 2003) within Europe, although welcome, are often not standardised and are unregulated. As a result some of these roles involve little more than the performance of junior doctors tasks.

This point was highlighted by a leading cardiac nurse/academic, Thompson (2002), who stated that many new roles of cardiac nurses 'have developed organically ... without any systematic planning or evaluation'. He also highlighted that 'there is a danger that [in these roles] nurses focus solely on particular aspects of medical treatment rather than focus on the totality of patient care'. He suggests that current evaluation of many of these roles indicates that they pay little attention to the 'important contextual factors' such as the person and environment.

Nursing has long been associated with the use of rituals and tradition, and although these have declined in many areas of nursing they still prevail (Riegel et al. 1996, Jacobson 2000, Strange 2001). There are a variety of reasons for this – lack of autonomy, lack of knowledge, hierarchical systems and avoidance measures, to name but a few. Little consensus exists regarding their exact origin, however, there is consensus that nursing needs to move away from these traditional operating frameworks towards evidence-informed nursing.

Evidence-informed nursing is 'the integration of professional judgement and research evidence' (McSherry et al. 2002: 3). It requires nurses to be 'knowledgeable doers' and have a 'systematic approach to providing nursing care' (McSherry et al. 2002: 3). Nurse theorists have long advocated for the use of nursing theory to inform a systematic approach to nursing care. Nursing theory offers research-derived evidence to inform the nursing knowledge base (Fawcett 2003). Stewart (2002) suggests that nurses in general and cardiovascular nurses in particular need to begin to generate new theory to inform practice.

Nursing theory offers nursing a distinct scientific knowledge base to guide practice. Without the use of nursing theory to guide practice, the work of the nurse may be oversimplified. In addition, nursing in some situations may appear as a discrete set of tasks or orders, thus under-estimating the complexity of the role. Given the increasingly medical aspects of some cardiac nursing roles as described by Thompson (2002), it is time therefore to consider the potential contribution of nursing theory to coronary care nursing.

There is considerable discussion and debate, within the nursing literature with regard to the usefulness of nursing theory to inform nursing practice. Fawcett (1999) expressed concern with today's nursing practice, suggesting that there is little evidence of nursing theory occupying what she describes as its true position as the central tenet of nursing practice. The fact is supported anecdotally in coronary care practice, where there is lack of consistency of both use and application of nursing theory.

Fawcett (1999) and Alligood (2002a) both strongly advocate that nurses base their practice upon nursing theory. Fawcett (1999) suggests that 'It has become increasingly clear to [her] that the discipline of nursing can survive if, and only if, we end our romance with medical science and the conceptual frameworks and theories of non-nursing disciplines'.

Fawcett (1999) would like all nurses to 'embrace' nursing theory and conceptual models to ensure survival of the discipline. The author recommends that all nurses must 'fall in love with nursing science now and develop a passion for the destiny of the discipline of nursing'. Conversely, Cormack and Reynolds (1992: 1473) suggested that the use of conceptual models and theory 'provides no more than a pseudo-scientific respectability'.

Despite Fawcett's (1999) and Alligood's (2002a) commitment to the development of nursing practice through nursing theory and conceptual model use, there is opposition within nursing to this view. Rawnsley (1999) in response to Fawcett's paper, rejected the notion of a purist knowledge base for nursing in favour of a more inclusive approach to nursing that draws on many areas of knowledge other than nursing. Similarly, Heath (1998) highlighted that many theorists have become preoccupied with the role of theory development in raising nursing's professional status rather than concentrating on what is best for the patient. Heath (1998) dismissed Fawcett's views regarding the need for a distinct body of knowledge to guide nursing and develop the discipline, as extreme. Much criticism of nursing theory and conceptual models of nursing also emanates from scholars who hold post-modern views (Timmins 2002).

The debate continues, however, from a practising nurse's perspective. Current evidence suggests that the use of theories and conceptual models of nursing may be a useful adjunct to practice and therefore should be embraced. Their development and use for cardiac nursing is also advocated (Fawcett et al. 1992, Stewart 2002, Timmins 2002).

The development of nursing knowledge has been a prevalent theme in the nursing literature for the past 30 years. Prior to the gradual development of nursing theory and conceptual models in the USA in the 1950s, Alligood (2002a) suggests that nursing practice was based on principles and traditions passed on through apprenticeship education and common-sense wisdom that came with years of experience. Although some nurse leaders aspired for nursing to develop as a profession and an academic discipline, 'nursing practice continued to reflect vocational heritage more than professional vision' (Alligood and Marriner-Tomey 2002a: 5). The latter have suggested that theory development in the USA has contributed to the transition of nursing from vocation to profession.

Although the USA has been largely responsible for theory development within nursing, it is recognised that scholarly work came from within Europe as evidenced by the plethora of nursing journals disseminating the research endeavours of many countries. Alligood (2002a) suggested that it is difficult to compare theory development within Europe to the USA. From an academic perspective, Europe has integrated nurse education into university settings less universally and at a slower pace than in the USA. As nursing schools within Europe began to formalise links with third-level institutes from the 1960s, nurses holding doctorate degrees were in the minority. This embryonic nature of postgraduate development of the profession as a whole has the effect of limiting scholarly activity (Treacy and Hyde 1999). The slow development of nursing science within Europe was highlighted by Evers (2002) suggesting difficulty with transference of American knowledge due to language and lack of empirical testing of American theories of nursing.

Despite the relative naivety of European nurses in theoretical and empirical development and the difficulties noted by Evers (2002), the American perspective on the profession of nursing and its theoretical base has been readily embraced in many areas. The work of many American theorists has been translated into several languages, and theories emanating from the USA are widely used throughout Europe (Fawcett 1995).

One theory of nursing developed in Edinburgh and forming the basis for the Roper-Logan-Tierney (RLT) model of nursing (Roper et al. 1980, 1985, 1990, 1996) is widely used throughout the UK and Ireland. Its recognition and inclusion in one recent text (Alligood and Marriner-Tomey 2002b) may indicate growing recognition by the USA of the presence of theory emanating from outside.

What is nursing theory?

Florence Nightingale (1820–1910), who laid the foundations of theoretical development in nursing, suggested that 'the most important practical lesson that can be
given to nurses is to teach them what to observe, how to observe, [and] what symptoms indicate improvement' (Nightingale 1992: 59), thus indicating the importance
then, as now, of a systematic and methodical approach to nursing care. She
described how patients who had a lot of information to give would provide little to
the nurse if the questioning technique was poor and unfocused. She went on to
describe 'how few there are who, by five or six pointed questions, can elicit the
whole case and get accurately to know and to be able to report where the patient is'
(Nightingale 1992: 61). Observation features highly in her writings and she suggests
careful and detailed observation with use of directive questioning can lead to appropriate diagnosis. This notion of guiding nurses' observation towards accurate diagnosis underpins much of today's nursing theory.

Nightingale (1992) also argued that nursing had a distinct function outside of
medicine in the observation and treatment of patients, prevention of disease and
evaluation of care. These words were written in a less sophisticated healthcare
environment; however, discerning what constitutes nursing and the notion that
nursing is more than the administration of medical orders are themes that permeate
the text, and have occupied nurse theorists for decades.

One prime motivator for the development of nursing theory in recent decades is
the belief that, although nurses work in parallel with many other healthcare professionals, they assess, plan, implement and evaluate care in their own right. Using
nursing theory to guide this process provides a suitable theoretical framework with
which to conceptualise, describe and inform the unique contribution of the nurse in
healthcare settings.

The complexity of contemporary nursing practice requires a systematic approach
that complies with current trends of patient-centred care. Application of theoretical
works to nursing practice serves to clarify the nurse's function in nursing situations
and provides a rationale for nursing actions. It also offers a unique perspective of
the patient that is holistic and not disease focused. The use of a conceptual model
prescribes a systematic approach to care based on sound theoretical principles, with
particular emphasis on assessment, planning, implementing and evaluation of care.
However, there are difficulties with the understanding and application of these concepts in practice.

Confusion exists with regard to differentiating between conceptual models and
theory (Fawcett 1995). The terms are often used interchangeably, and while many
theorists outline both a theory and a conceptual model, significant differences exist
in the definition and understanding of both (Fawcett 1995).

Practising nurses are most familiar with the use of conceptual models. These are
one component of what Fawcett (1995) termed a structural hierarchy of nursing
knowledge. Fawcett's (1989, 1993, 1995) work was pivotal in developing nursing's
understanding of conceptual models. This important contribution was acknowledged by Alligood who suggested that Fawcett developed 'a paradigm explanation
of the interconnectedness of the various nursing theoretical works ... which began
to clarify different levels of abstraction ...' (2002a: 8).

Fawcett (1995) stated that conceptual models form the fourth component in a hierarchy; the first component is the metaparadigm, the second is philosophy, the third is theory and the fourth is conceptual models (Box 1.1). The metaparadigm outlines global concepts that identify what phenomena are of interest to any discipline. This is the most abstract level of knowledge in the hierarchy. It specifies the main concepts that encompass the subject matter and the scope of the discipline. In nursing, these are *the person, the environment, health* and *nursing* (Alligood and Marriner-Tomey 2002c).

These concepts form the four central areas of interest to nursing (Fawcett 1995). The person is the receiver of care, including individuals, families and communities. The environment is the person's family, physical surroundings and the healthcare setting. Health is the 'person's state of well being ...' (Fawcett 1995: 7). Nursing is that which is done by nurses for the patient.

The concepts of a metaparadigm are extremely broad. They serve to represent the views within a discipline, and distinguish a domain which is very different from that of other disciplines, but its purpose is not to provide direct guidance to practice (Fawcett 1995).

Philosophy is the second component in the structural hierarchy of contemporary nursing knowledge (Fawcett 1995). It may be defined as a statement of beliefs and values (Kim 1983). The path from the metaparadigm of the discipline to philosophy is non-linear, i.e. philosophy does not follow directly in line from the metaparadigm, and does not directly precede conceptual models. Rather a cyclical relationship exists. The metaparadigm identifies areas about which philosophical claims are made. The unique focus and context of each conceptual model then reflects the underlying philosophy (Fawcett 1995).

The next component in the structural hierarchy of nursing knowledge is theory. Theory is a concept devised for a particular purpose. In nursing this purpose goes beyond description to theory that informs the nursing situation. Theory, although abstract, is capable of being translated into reality. Theory is a proposed structure that shapes and guides reality. This structure is made up of things and situations that constitute the theory (Dickoff and James 1968).

Theories that are broadest in scope are called grand theories. These are made up of rather abstract and general concepts and propositions that cannot be generated or tested empirically. Middle-range theories are narrower in scope and contain a limited number of concepts which are empirically measurable. Middle-range theories are the least abstract level of theoretical knowledge because they include details specific to nursing practice, such as patient condition (Alligood and Marriner-Tomey

---

Box 1.1 The nursing knowledge hierarchy

- Metaparadigm
- Philosophy
- Theory
- Conceptual models

Adapted from Fawcett, J. (1995) *Analysis and Evaluation of Conceptual Models of Nursing,* 3rd edn. Philadelphia: F.A. Davies.

2002a). Theories are described as either unique or borrowed. The latter are borrowed from other disciplines rather than developed exclusively for nursing.

The final component in the structural hierarchy is conceptual models of nursing. These provide explanations of nursing. They identify the purpose and scope of nursing and provide frameworks recording nursing actions and effects (Fawcett 1995) and frameworks for systematic approaches to nursing care. Each conceptual model provides a unique direction to nursing practice.

Advocates of conceptual-model-based practice consider models useful adjuncts to guide complex nursing situations (Bush 1997). It is also suggested that the demands of the healthcare environment are such that nurses often do not have the time to investigate every aspect of a patient's situation and that conceptual models provide a framework that allows for prioritisation in assessment and care planning (Raudonis and Gayle 1997). This is consistent with Nightingale's (1992) call for astute observation by nurses to prevent misdiagnosis and missing important patient cues.

It is also argued that models facilitate nursing practice becoming more logical and less reliant on tradition and intuition: there is a systematic rather than a routine approach to care. Nursing care delivery becomes more consistent and precise with their use (Alligood 2002b). Rather than each nurse using their own experience and ideas about the world to guide their practice, the suggested framework, philosophy and theories inherent in each model guides them (Raudonis and Gayle 1997). Nightingale (1992) also advocated a structured approach to patient assessment, rather than relying on personal and traditional practices.

Nursing is a relatively new discipline and, although significant theoretical development has taken place over the past 30 years, nursing knowledge is now at a crossroads. To complete the cycle of theory development, practical application and testing is essential. In order for nursing knowledge to make a difference, it must be used in practice settings. Nursing is entering a new era, according to Alligood (2002a) – theory utilisation – where nurses begin to use and research nursing theory in practice settings. This may add the crucial dimension that the current theory development cycle requires, thus narrowing the hiatus that exists at present between theory and practice in some areas (Wood and Alligood 2002).

Although knowledge development emanates from the testing of theories in the practice setting, conceptual model use is also crucial to this phase of nursing knowledge development. Fawcett (1999) suggested that the latter is not only a 'hallmark of success in nursing' but would ensure the 'survival of nursing as a discipline', which she fears, is in danger of extinction (Fawcett 2000). There are many, including Fawcett (1995, 1999, 2000) who argue that the recognition of nursing as a distinct discipline and a profession is dependent on ensuring that nursing practice has a sound theoretical base.

While utilisation is important, it is also important to take nursing knowledge development one step further by evaluating benefits to patients, staff and nursing situations. A gap exists in this particular aspect of nursing knowledge that is evident in the literature on the topic.

The RLT conceptual model for example has professed benefits such as developing nursing curricula and improved documentation and individualised care (Tierney 1998). However, by the admission of one of the co-authors, there is limited empirical evidence in existence supporting the effects of RLT use on patient outcomes (Tierney 1998). Griffiths (1998), Mason (1999) and Murphy et al. (2000), who all examined the use of RLT in a variety of nursing situations, revealed that it did little to inform practice and the associated documentation was cumbersome.

Orem's Self Care Deficit Nursing Theory (SCDNT) (Orem 2001), although purported to be one of the most widely used theories in practice (Berbiglia 2002), also has empirical deficits. While the literature abounds with practical application of Orem's conceptual model, few empirical studies have examined SCDNT in practice (Spearman et al. 1993, Taylor et al. 2000). Many studies identified both by Spearman et al. (1993) and Taylor et al. (2000) in their reviews, revealed that while the SCDNT was often used as an organising framework or a component of the study its use was so limited that it did little to advance nursing knowledge in this area.

Spearman et al. (1993) found that, while many studies used Orem's SCDNT as a basis for research, the majority (87%) had minimal or insufficient use of theory. Only four studies (13%) were categorised as adequately using theory. Similarly, Taylor et al. (2000) highlighted that the studies were descriptive in nature; only one experimental study was identified. Most studies focused on further description of the theory and only few studies examined theory from a practice perspective.

This may be a reflection of the embryonic stage of theory development within nursing. According to Toulmin's (1972) four-stage framework, nursing theory evolution is not complete. In the first stage, the discipline identifies its own body of knowledge, areas of concern, methods and goals in a slow developmental fashion. This is certainly evident in nursing from the existing hierarchy of nursing knowledge. Stage two involves the filtering of ideas and concepts with rejection and retention of ideas as appropriate with those fitting the discipline surviving over time. Nursing theory has undergone limited empirical testing and refinement, with scepticism evident in the discipline to its usefulness and place in nursing. The third phase involves adaptation of theory by the discipline in an environment of debate, critique and innovation. The extent to which this has taken place is debatable. Although some individual theories and conceptual models have been adapted and developed, much exising theory remains irrelevant and obscure to nurses in practice. Some perceive that this is due to a failure to develop theories that are appropriate to the everyday needs of nursing practice. In the final phase, ideas, concepts and theories that are most useful in meeting the local demands are selected by the discipline for use. Although Meleis (1997) rejects the notion that the development of nursing knowledge could or should follow an evolutionary course, a gap exists between theory development and use of theory in practice (Bush 1997).

Recognition that current scepticism about nursing theory and conceptual model use in nursing is a natural development that concurs with stage two of Toulmin's (1972) framework of concept evolution may pave the way for movement towards adaptation and critical debate on the topic prior to the final utilisation phase. Stewart (2002) recognised that nursing is struggling with its theoretical foundation and suggests that it is time for 'rigorous debate and constructive criticism within our profession . . . it is time for us to shrug off our comfortable apathy and become more engaged'. Although Alligood (2002a) suggested that we are entering the utilisation phase, from a European perspective, there is time for more critical discussion, debate and adaptation prior to this event.

In today's ever-changing complex coronary care environment, nurses require a high level of skills. The demands of coronary care require practitioners to adopt thoughtful insightful practices. These attributes are key components of what is termed as *critical practice* (Brechin 2000: 26). Critical practice is firmly enshrined in the practice domain. Building upon the work of Barnett, Brechin (2000) suggested that inherent domains of critical practice are critical analysis, critical action and critical reflexivity. They suggest that health professionals require all three skills to meet the challenges of a practice that is filled with uncertainty (Brechin 2000). *Critical analysis* requires on-going enquiry and analysis. Rather than simply relying upon prior knowledge and practices the practitioner *evaluates* their relevance.

As an alternative to the pursuit of a new theory for cardiovascular nursing as suggested by Stewart (2002), critical practice challenges nurses to evaluate current knowledge and theory (critical analysis), question personal values and assumptions (critical reflexivity) and use these to inform a sound skill base (critical action). Nurses are challenged therefore to question the extent to which current nursing knowledge informs practice.

Using nursing knowledge to inform nursing practice

The potential of knowledge development within nursing to raise the professional profile of nursing is a predominant theme in the literature. However, the ability for this knowledge to translate into real benefits in practice is debatable. In addition, there is evidence of reluctance to apply nursing theory and conceptual models in practice.

The notion of nursing theory is clearly a product of the USA and it often elicits debate concerning the relevance and usefulness of theory in and for nursing in Europe (Riley et al. 2003). Timpson (1996: 1030) suggests that 'nursing theory has a reputation for abstraction, even irrelevance, in the minds of many practitioners. A case very much of art for art's sake'.

One possible reason for reluctance to apply theory in practice is the questionable potential of abstract theories to guide what is primarily a practical discipline. Nurses in practice also often fail to see where theory can guide and improve practice when, on a day-to-day basis, nursing frequently meets the goals of patient care without the use of a clearly defined theory.

This latter success hypothetically emanates from nurses operating from their own personal knowledge base, using it as a frame of reference for practice (Johnson 1987, Ellis 1989). Despite the purported success with this approach Ellis (1989) suggested that the result is the application of 'imperfectly articulated intuitive knowledge'. While some level of intuition is clearly important for nursing practice (Johnson 1987, Ellis 1989) Timpson (1996) suggests that the absence of a sound theoretical base can potentially reduce nursing 'to the domain of the common-sense'.

Clearly, the lack of a sound theoretical base has the potential to undermine the professionalism that many have been striving for many years to achieve. However, for theory to be widely accepted by nurses, its applicability and relevance to practice must be clear. In the early stages of theory development, Dickoff and James (1968) and Ellis (1968) stated that theory *must* be useful for and be able to guide nursing practice.

Recent studies confirm the difficulty that nurses have with the application of conceptual models in practice. Griffiths (1998) examined the effects of two conceptual models of nursing on nurses' descriptions of patients' problems. The findings revealed that when describing patients' problems there was little evidence of application of the two models. Information was often not committed to written record but rather stored 'in the memory of the nurses', which Griffiths (1998) suggested was problematic as 'essential information was often only lodged in the nurse's head, and thus subject to loss'.

Similarly, Murphy et al. (2000) revealed that nursing staff were ambivalent towards the use of conceptual-model-based care plans. This study examined whether or not the RLT conceptual model was a suitable model for directing nursing care for clients with mental illness in an Irish setting. The findings revealed that the model had guided assessment and interventions in very few cases. Most evaluations of identified goals were not completed. Nearly all care plans revealed under-utilisation of the model. The study indicated a lack of consistent and appropriate use of the model.

These findings echo Mason's (1999) UK study into the use of care plans with the RLT conceptual model. Completing care plans was a burden to busy staff and did little to contribute to planning or evaluating care. Consistent with Griffiths' (1998) study, staff relied on verbal reports rather than the care plans. Most nurses in the study were 'keen to voice their dislike of care plans', describing them in derogatory terms.

Negative views of conceptual models in practice may be compounded by a view that most nursing theories and conceptual models profess universal application. Contemporary views are that a careful selection process takes place so the model chosen reflects the values and beliefs of the nurses using it. In addition, where lack of control in implementation is perceived, which was the case in Mason's (1999) study, there is a lack of trust and ownership of the model. In the past, managers often imposed models of nursing upon nurses. While this impetus may have been well intended from a management perspective, this top-down approach is very likely to result in resistance.

Systematic selection of conceptual models for practice is endorsed by many authors (Mason and Chandley 1992, Bush 1997, Lister 1997). Bush suggests that it is the responsibility of practising nurses to analyse conceptual models to ascertain their potential benefits and contribution to practice.

Selection of a conceptual model of nursing for use in the coronary care unit

Many areas of practice lack consensus regarding the use of models, indeed, Fawcett et al. (1992) noted that application of conceptual models to critical care nursing has been addressed by few authors with no consensus emerging as to one best fit.

What is clear from the literature is that conceptual-based nursing in the clinical area requires a systematic process of selection and adoption. Rather than prescribing models for use, this approach allows nurses to make their own choice, depending on individual practice circumstances. This is consistent with the notion of critical practice. Providing nurses with a quick solution of the best-fit model may reduce model use to a series of tasks (such as documentation, as revealed in many studies), which totally contradicts the whole ethos of conceptual model-based care. Or the model may exist on paper but not reflect the reality of practice (Griffiths 1998). Indeed, Mason and Chandley's (1992) qualitative exploration of model (unidentified) use by nurses described a 'hyperreality', where the model had a camouflage quality that did not reflect reality. Empowering nurses to critically evaluate conceptual models for practice and adapt them for use in practice is the only means of these concepts being truly accepted by nurses and used in practice.

In one paper, Fawcett et al. (1992) suggested that selection of conceptual models of nursing may be guided by individual patient need, rather than subscribing to the notion that one model fits all. However, the practicalities of implementing individualised care according to the most suitable model for each patient are fraught with difficulty. Indeed, Fawcett (1995) later suggested that it is best for the whole healthcare institute to adopt one conceptual model to avoid confusion.

Fawcett (1995) outlined a more generalised approach to the implementation of conceptual-model-based nursing, recommending an eight-stage approach to the selection process. The first phase involves articulating a vision. The second phase entails forming a group to determine feasibility of implementation. This may include nurses who may have a particular interest in this area or nursing managers who require and change in practice in this area. If the implementation appears to be feasible, the third phase begins involving forming a planning group and devising long-term goals. Key nursing personnel from the clinical arena need to be involved at this stage. The fourth phase entails a review of documents that serve as a base for nursing practice, including the mission statement and philosophy (Fawcett, 1995). In the fifth phase, staff choose a conceptual model. Fawcett (1995) suggests that this phase should proceed through four main steps (Box 1.2).

Fawcett (1995) also suggested that it is essential that this fifth phase involves comparing various conceptual models to the beliefs and values of healthcare institutes. She recommended that education of nursing staff is crucial and this constitutes the sixth phase. In phase seven, Fawcett suggested that a pilot scheme should be introduced, whereby certain clinical areas are chosen to adopt the process for a

---

Box 1.2 The process for choosing a conceptual model of nursing for use in the healthcare setting

1. Analyse and evaluate several conceptual models of nursing
2. Compare the content of each conceptual model with the mission statement of the healthcare institute to determine if the model is appropriate for use with the population of care recipients served
3. Determine if the philosophy that underpins each model is congruent with the philosophy of the nursing department
4. Select the conceptual model that most closely matches the mission of the healthcare institute and the philosophy of the nursing department

Adapted from Fawcett, J. (1995) *Analysis and Evaluation of Conceptual Models of Nursing*, 3rd edn. Philadelphia: F.A. Davies.

designated period. This phase is essential to deal with any initial problems that may arise. The final phase (eight), is widespread adoption of the conceptual-model-based nursing practice throughout the healthcare setting.

Using a systematic approach as outlined above to the selection and adoption of a conceptual model for nursing care is crucial to success in practice. Empirical and anecdotal evidence suggests that where conceptual-model-based practice is imposed upon staff with little consultation, the result is limited use of the model in practice. A systematic approach allows nursing staff in the clinical area to have ownership of the project and this is likely to yield successful adaptation. This has been demonstrated in some nursing areas (see McClune and Franklin 1987, Sutcliffe 1994 and Graeme 2000).

Several papers have addressed conceptual model selection; these often refer to selection *and* subsequent adaptation of models. Although adapting models for use in practice is not a concept that has received much attention in American-based theoretical literature, there is growing interest in the UK towards adapting models at the local level. Roper et al. (2001) stated that their model might be adapted for use in the practice setting.

The Mead model (Sutcliffe 1994) is commonly referred to when considering models for use in critical care settings. It is an adaptation of the RLT model developed on Mead Ward, St Thomas's Hospital, London (McClune and Franklin 1987). Sutcliffe (1994) reported how this model was selected for use in the Royal Brompton Hospital's intensive care unit (ICU) and renamed the Mead model. Sutcliffe's paper reports a good example of staff working together to develop a shared philosophy and using this to inform selection of model of nursing. An audit revealed that the previous model in use was not congruent with the philosophy of the unit and therefore was disregarded by many staff in the course of their duties. Sutcliffe (1994) described how most nurses were instead using their own personal philosophies and models to guide and direct patient care. Sutcliffe (1994) felt that this resulted in care being given in a very individualised manner that caused confusion, particularly for nursing students and new staff.

Sutcliffe's (1994) first task was to develop a nursing philosophy for the unit. This corresponds with Fawcett's (1995) first step in utilisation, creating a vision of nursing. A collaborate approach was used, whereby organised staff meetings were conducted on the unit at convenient times. The attitudes, beliefs and values of the staff were explored and articulated through brainstorming sessions and methods of anonymously presenting opinions. The attitudes, values and beliefs identified (Box 1.3) were incorporated into a unit philosophy by the staff during a series of meetings.

Once the philosophy was outlined, Sutcliffe (1994) was confident that the nurses had embraced the notion of a shared philosophy and that linking theory to practice would be a natural progression. The author was surprised and pleased by the level of staff empowerment, as they went on to develop a 'nursing model action plan', without further outside assistance. This action is congruent with Fawcett's (1995) third phase of utilisation, the formation of a planning committee and outlining long-term goals.

The staff outlined their goals for practice (Box 1.4) and began a search for a suitable model. This process involved individuals and groups critically analysing selected models and presenting the results to staff in the department. Following this,

---

Box 1.3 Attitudes, values and beliefs of the critical care nursing team as identified by staff at the Royal Brompton Hospital ICU (1994)

- Attitudes of a critical care nurse
  Caring
  Technically competent
  Confident
  Professional
  Educated

- Values of the critical care team
  The individual
  The family
  The nurse
  Knowledge and skills
  Quality of life
  Caring
  Technically competent
  Confident

- Beliefs of the critical care team
  Nursing is unique and holistic
  Individuals have the right to a high quality of life
  Critical care nursing requires interpersonal, academic and technical skills
  Education is a key element

Adapted from Sutcliffe, L. (1994) Philosophy and models in critical care nursing. *Intensive and Critical Care Nursing* 10: 212–221.

Box 1.4 Goals for practice identified by staff at the Brompton ICU (1994)

- Promoting independence in the patient
- Dignified death
- Preventing problems
- Involvement of the family

Adapted from Sutcliffe, L. (1994) Philosophy and models in critical care nursing. *Intensive and Critical Care Nursing* 10: 212–221.

---

in-depth discussions between the staff regarding the suitability of a variety of models took place. In the end the staff settled on RLT as adapted in the Mead model. The staff felt that the RLT model in its original format did not deal specifically enough with the physical aspects of care, which are a feature of critical care units, but could identify with the adaptations. They perceived, however, that the family did not receive enough attention in either the RLT or the Mead model so in their use of the model they placed the family (and the individual within) at the centre. In addition, another area that caused concern was the 'rather loose guidelines for assessing the individual – especially general headings physical. Patients admitted to the critical care area generally have physical needs that take priority.

Although the ability to assess these needs was well developed in many experienced critical care nurses, the Brompton hospital received many novice nurses so it was felt that it was necessary to have clear guidelines to provide direction. They therefore used prompts within each assessment category [Activity of Daily Living (AL)] to allow for an in-depth assessment of each area. The staff have been using the adapted model for more than a year and have found it to be 'very successful in enabling us [them] to put into action the beliefs identified in the unit philosophy' (Sutcliffe 1994). However, as reported frequently in other studies, they found the documentation time-consuming.

A crucial stage in the selection process is matching the values inherent in the model with values of the nursing situations. Alligood (2002b) suggests, the writing of a brief philosophy of nursing in the initial selection stage is useful and serves to clarify beliefs and values held by nurses in the area. Once beliefs are clarified a survey of the definitions of person, environment, health and nursing within various nursing models and theories can be carried out. A model may then be selected that is congruent with these beliefs. When in use it can be tailored 'to the special aspects of your art of nursing' (Alligood 2002b: 57).

Graeme (2000) also used this process and outlined the selection of a conceptual model for a newly opened 18-bedded palliative care unit. The whole nursing team was involved in devising the model and patients were involved in evaluation. The staff initially decided on their collective philosophy of care, based on the beliefs and values of the nursing team. Then they began a search for a suitable model but 'no off-the-shelf model seemed to fit'. They opted for an eclectic selection and devised the 'Shipley model' (Graeme 2000).

Both Sutcliffe's (1994) and Graeme's (2000) papers outline a thoughtful and inclusive approach to the implementation of conceptual-model-based practice. Their particular emphasis on staff inclusion and identification of core beliefs, values and philosophies is congruent with Fawcett's (1995) guidelines. The result was successful adoption of models in practice. The education of the staff appeared to be a dynamic component of the process, rather than a formalised education structure. The latter would need to be considered by coronary care units considering model implementation or development, as education is fundamental to the process. In addition, the use of a pilot to test the model would help to familiarise staff and identify problems early before full implementation. Critical evaluation and analysis of conceptual models needs consideration.

Fawcett (1995) suggested that analysis and evaluation of conceptual models is an essential component of the selection process. Both Sutcliffe (1994) and Graeme (2000) highlight the failure of conceptual models to fully address their needs, however, the extent to which they performed a critical analysis of the models is unclear. Both authors were strongly guided by the beliefs and values of the staff in the units, which is an integral component of implementation (Fawcett 1995). However, of equal value in the process is the identification of potential conceptual models and subsequent critical analysis to reveal particular strengths and weakness. This is termed analysis and evaluation by Fawcett (1995) (these terms are used interchangeably with critical analysis and critical appraisal). Several frameworks to support this analysis are present in both nursing theory texts and papers on the topic.

Critical appraisal of conceptual models

Robinson (1993) suggested that nursing theories and models should not be adopted uncritically, as they may not be culturally applicable or easily adaptable. It is important that coronary care nurses adopt systems for evaluating conceptual nursing models. Critical thinking is an essential competency of nursing that requires nurses to challenge assumptions, consider context and use reflective scepticism (Brookfield 1987). Critical thinking underpins many of the components of critical practice (Brechin 2000) and ensures the adoption of a critical approach not only to the implementation but also to the appraisal of conceptual models.

In the past conceptual models were often adopted uncritically by nurses in practice with resultant apathy regarding use when they did not operationalise well. Critical appraisal is an essential step in the process of implementing conceptual-model-based practice. Use of systematic frameworks to guide this process is a recurring theme in the literature, with most theoretical texts offering advice in this area.

Cormack and Reynolds (1992) outlined one such framework for evaluating the clinical and practical utility of models used by nurses. They suggested that nurses should evaluate the possible contribution of the model to practice, before selecting it for use. They present a set of criteria that nurses can use to evaluate a model in order to establish its value in the clinical setting (Box 1.5).

Box 1.5 Criteria for evaluating the clinical and practical utility of conceptual models of nursing

- Is the conceptual model clearly understood by nurses?
- Is the scope of the conceptual model clearly delineated?
- Does the conceptual model outline an approach that is specific to nurses and nursing?
- Is the conceptual model based on tested and accepted theory?
- Is the conceptual model valid and reliable?
- Is the conceptual model geographically portable?
- Does the conceptual model assist with the identification of the range of human responses to actual or potential health problems?
- Does the conceptual model provide an explanation for common human responses to health problems experienced by individuals?
- Does the conceptual model enable nurses to identify nursing interventions?
- Does the conceptual model specify the desired outcome of nursing interventions?
- Does the conceptual model comply with accepted ethical standards in nursing?

Adapted from Cormack, D.F.S. and Reynolds, W. (1992) Criteria for evaluating the clinical and practical utility of models used by nurses. *Journal of Advanced Nursing* 17: 1472–1478.

Using these questions to examine the potential benefits of conceptual-model-based practice can be quite helpful to nurses in the coronary care unit. It is often difficult to assess the strengths and weaknesses of conceptual models without the assistance of a formalised structure. This framework enables the nurse to make judgements about the conceptual model without over-reliance on anecdotal evidence. It allows for an informed and balanced judgement regarding the crucial components of a conceptual model. Consistent with other suggested frameworks identified in the literature, it does not provide strict guidance, such as scoring system, to interpret the responses but leaves interpretation open to the user. While this approach may be criticised for lack of direction it does allow the judgement regarding the importance of each item to be worked out at a local level.

Many writers express the difficulty nurses experience with the understanding of conceptual models and Cormack and Reynolds (1992) suggest that the model should be easy to understand. This guideline empowers nurses to reject a conceptual model if its underlying theory, philosophy and methodology are incoherent to the nurses in the area. They suggest that if the average nurse does not understand it then the model will be of limited value in practice. The RLT model (Roper et al. 1980, 1985, 1990, 1996), which was used extensively in Europe in the 1980s and 1990s, was noted to be easily understood (Marriner-Tomey 2000) – one reason, perhaps, for its relative popularity.

Cormack and Reynolds (1992) also state that the scope of the model should be clearly delineated. It should be clear whether or not the model is applicable to the particular clinical setting and if it could meet the needs of the specific patient group. Most conceptual models claim generalisability across settings and do not explicitly recommend its use in particular settings. However, examination of the theoretical underpinnings of the model, including its definition of nursing, the environment, health and the individual, should be clear. This information may guide clinicians as to the suitability for use in particular settings. Another route for exploration is to search for literature that examines or uses the conceptual model; this may give an indication of its scope in a particular area. Many textbooks on conceptual models, such as Alligood and Marriner-Tomey (2002b) and Fawcett (1995), outline studies and other literature in which particular conceptual models have been utilised and these may also serve as a guide.

Cormack and Reynolds (1992) suggest that regardless of whether the model is unique to nursing or borrowed from another discipline it should inform clinicians in a manner that is unique to nursing. Cormack and Reynolds (1992) also stated that the model should contain specific information regarding its reliability and validity to inform practitioners. This is not always contained within primary sources; however, evaluation issues such as these and many others are dealt with in depth by many exceptional texts on the topic, such as Fawcett (1995), Meleis (1997) and Alligood and Marriner-Tomey (2002b).

Cormack and Reynolds (1992) view the issue of geographical portability as a serious one. They recognise that most models of nursing have emanated from the USA and have been globally applied to nursing situations. They suggest that it is therefore essential to consider the transferability of concepts, language and methodology, and to carefully assess usefulness in the particular setting from a cultural perspective before embarking on the conceptual model. Evers (2002) suggested that the difficulty with transferring language contributed to stifling nursing theory development in Europe. This point was clearly highlighted by Shamsudin (2002), who used a grounded theory approach to the adaptation of a conceptual model of nursing to Malyasian nursing practice.

Cormack and Reynolds (1992) also suggested that a model should easily assist the nurse to identify a patient's problems, provide an explanation for human responses, enable nurses to identify nursing intervention, and specify the potential outcome of care. The model should also allow nurses to use it within the constraints and responsibilities of their practice and it should comply with ethical principles in nursing. The extent to which the conceptual model is capable of this is dependent on the particular context and the views of the nurses. It is also dependent on the decision makers having an accurate knowledge of the inherent properties of the conceptual model, which facilitates an informed judgement.

Nursing staff in contemporary coronary care units often operate in high-pressure environments with high patient turnover and significant patient morbidity. Current emphasis on providing evidence-based care encourages nurses to question the evidence that informs their practice. While there are not many empirical studies supporting conceptual-model-based practice, there is sufficient evidence to convince many of their usefulness in practice and their potential benefits to patients, nurse satisfaction, delivery of nursing services and the development of the profession.

Using evidence in practice involves the integration of professional judgement and empirical evidence (McSherry et al. 2002). Conceptual-model-based practice, which has been a feature of Western nursing for the last three decades, now requires a greater integration of professional judgement with the existing evidence to evaluate the usefulness of conceptual models in the coronary care unit. This requires reflection on current practice, the use of key texts on the topic, such as Fawcett (1995), Meleis (1997) and Alligood and Marriner-Tomey (2002b), and the use of systematic evaluative frameworks, such as Cormack and Reynolds (1985) or those outlined in the preceding textbooks. Where conceptual models are in current use, it may be useful to evaluate their effectiveness. The process outlined for selecting a model can be adapted to aid staff in developing current models in a local setting. However, given the complexity of today's healthcare environment, it is becoming increasingly important that nurses within particular areas all operate from a similar frame of reference.

The use of conceptual-model-based nursing provides frameworks that guide nurses in the assessment, planning, implementation, and evaluation of patient care. Their use in coronary care units may guide nurses to conceptualise and prioritise observations and care. In addition, this approach reflects a dimension of care that is distinctly nursing. While nursing practice is inextricably enmeshed in multidisciplinary practice, ensuring that patients receive not only consistent and coherent care, but also the best possible care, is reliant on outlining and operationalising the unique contribution nursing through the use of conceptual models to guide practice.

The nursing process (assess, plan, implement and evaluate) is often used to operationalise conceptual-model-based nursing. This is facilitated in practice by the use of documentation that guides the nurse in these areas. In order to demonstrate the use of a conceptual model in practice the following chapter focuses on planning nursing care using Orem's self-care deficit theory, providing examples of proposed documentation.

Summary and conclusions

The discipline of nursing is progressing from that of vocation to one of professional status in many countries. Nurses are highly valued by society and the individual practitioners' skill and artistry are an integral component to the dynamic of the practice setting. Nursing theory and conceptual model use are considerable attributes to this growing profession and, while conceptual model use is common in many areas of nursing practice, nurses need to develop a deeper understanding of its theoretical foundation and its potential usefulness to nursing situations. This is consistent with critical practice, which is a feature of contemporary nursing.

Whether conceptual model use is being considered for the first time, or reconsidered in a unit where model use exists, it is important to consider the fit between the model and the unit's philosophy. It is also important to involve the healthcare team in model selection to increase ownership and improve likelihood of success. It is also important to use a systematic approach and critically analyse the chosen model. In today's environment of the evidence base it is no longer acceptable to practice unquestioningly. While conceptual models of nursing undoubtedly have a strong empirical grounding, it remains the nurse's responsibility to question the evidence that informs particular model use. Blind acceptance of models in practice, can result in replacing new rituals for old. This is evident in many studies.

For conceptual model use to become a reality and make a difference to practice, nurses need to take ownership of the models, select an appropriate one for use, develop and adapt it locally if necessary and above all evaluate its usefulness and contribution to quality patient care using rigorous research.

References

Alligood, M.R. (2002a) The nature of knowledge needed for nursing practice. In: Alligood, M.R. and Marriner-Tomey, A. (eds) *Nursing Theory Utilisation & Application*. London: Mosby.

Alligood, M.R. (2002b) Models and theories: critical thinking structures. In: Alligood, M.R. and Marriner-Tomey, A. (eds) *Nursing Theory Utilisation & Application*. London: Mosby.

Alligood, M.R. and Marriner-Tomey, A. (2002a) Introduction to nursing theory: History, terminology, and analysis is practice. In: Alligood, M.R. and Marriner-Tomey, A. (eds) *Nursing Theorists and Their Work*, 5th edn. London: Mosby.

Alligood, M.R. and Marriner-Tomey, A. (2002b) (eds) *Nursing Theorists and Their Work*, 5th edn. London: Mosby.

Alligood, M.R. and Marriner-Tomey, A. (2002c) Significance of theory for nursing as a discipline. In: Alligood, M.R. and Marriner-Tomey, A. (eds) *Nursing Theorists and Their Work*, 5th edn. London: Mosby.

Berbiglia, V.A. (2002) Orem's Self-Care Deficit Nursing Theory in practice. In: Alligood, M.R. and Marriner-Tomey, A. (eds) *Nursing Theorists and Their Work*, 5th edn. London: Mosby.

Brechin, A. (2000) Introducing critical practice. In: Brechin, A., Brown, H. and Eby, M. (eds) *Critical Practice in Health and Social Care*. London: Sage Publications.

Brookfield, S.D. (1987) *Developing Critical Thinkers*. Milton Keynes: Open University Press.

Bush, H.A. (1997) Models for nursing. In: Nicoll, L.H. (ed) *Perspectives on Nursing Theory*, 3rd edn. New York: Lippincott.

Cormack, D.F.S. and Reynolds, W. (1992) Criteria for evaluating the clinical and practical utility of models used by nurses. *Journal of Advanced Nursing* 17: 1472–1478.

Dickoff, J. and James, P. (1968) A theory of theories: a position paper. *Nursing Research* 17(3): 197–203.

Ellis, R. (1968) Characteristics of significant theories. *Nursing Research* 17(3): 217–222.

Ellis, R. (1989) *Professional Competence and Quality Assurance in the Caring Professions.* London: Chapman Hall.

Evers, G. (2002) Developing nursing science in Europe. *Journal of Nursing Scholarship* 35(1): 9–13.

Fawcett, J. (1989) *Analysis and Evaluation of Conceptual Models of Nursing,* 2nd edn. Philadelphia: F.A. Davis.

Fawcett, J. (1993) *Analysis and Evaluation of Nursing Theories.* Philadelphia: F.A. Davis.

Fawcett, J. (1995) *Analysis and Evaluation of Conceptual Models of Nursing,* 3rd edn. Philadelphia: F.A. Davies.

Fawcett, J. (1999) The state of nursing science: hallmarks of the 20th and 21st centuries. *Nursing Science Quarterly* 12(4): 311–314.

Fawcett, J. (2000) The state of nursing science: where is the nursing in the science? *Theoria: Journal of Nursing Theory* 9(3): 3–10.

Fawcett, J. (2003) Orem's self-care deficit nursing theory: actual and potential sources for evidence-based practice. *Self-Care, Dependent-Care, and Nursing* 11(1): 11–16.

Fawcett, J., Archer, C.L., Becker, D., Brown, K.K., Gann, S., Wong, M.J. and Wurster, A.B. (1992) Guidelines for selecting a conceptual model of nursing: focus on the individual patient. *Dimensions of Critical Care Nursing* 11(5): 268–277.

Graeme, A. (2000) A post-modern nursing model. *Nursing Standard* 14(34): 40–42.

Griffiths, P. (1998) An investigation into the description of patients' problems by nurses using two different needs-based nursing models. *Journal of Advanced Nursing* 28(5): 969–977.

Heath, H. (1998) Paradigm dialogues and dogma: finding a place for research, nursing models and reflective practice. *Journal of Advanced Nursing* 28(2): 228–294.

Jacobson, A.F. (2000) Research utilization in nursing: the power of one. *Orthopedic Nursing* 19(6): 61–65.

Johnson, D.E. (1987) Evaluating conceptual models for use in critical care nursing practice. *Dimensions of Critical Care Nursing* 6: 195–197.

Kim, H.S. (1983) *The Nature of Theoretical Thinking in Nursing.* Connecticut: Appleton-Century Crofts.

Lister, P. (1997) The art of nursing in a 'postmodern' context. *Journal of Advanced Nursing* 25: 38–44.

Marriner-Tomey, A. (2000) Foreword. In: Roper, N., Logan, W.W. and Tierney, A.J. *The Roper Logan Tierney Model of Nursing Based on Activities of Living.* London: Churchill Livingstone.

Mason, C. (1999) Guide to practice or 'load of rubbish'? The influence of care plans on nursing practice in five clinical areas in Northern Ireland. *Journal of Advanced Nursing* 29(2): 380–387.

Mason, T. and Chandley, M (1992) Nursing models in a special hospital: cybernetics. Hyper-reality and beyond. *Journal of Advanced Nursing* 17: 1350–1354.

McClune, B. and Franklin, K. (1987) The Mead model for nursing – adapted from the Roper/Logan/Tierney model for nursing. *Intensive Care Nursing* 3: 97–103.

McSherry, R., Simmons, M. and Pearce, P. (2002) An introduction to evidence-informed nursing. In: McSherry, R., Simmons, M. and Pearce, P. (eds) *Evidence-Informed Nursing A Guide for Clinical Nurses.* London: Routledge.

Meleis, A.I. (1997) *Theoretical Nursing Development and Progress,* 3rd edn. New York: Lippincott.

Murphy, K., Cooney, A., Casey, D., Connor, M. O'Connor, J. and Dineen, B. (2000) The Roper, Logan and Tierney Model: perceptions and operationalization of the model in psychiatric nursing within one health board in Ireland. *Journal of Advanced Nursing*, 31(6): 1333–1341.

Nightingale, F. (1992) *Notes on Nursing: What It Is, and What It Is Not*, Commemorative edn. London: Lippincott Williams and Wilkins.

Orem, D.E. (1971, 1980, 1985, 1995, 2001) *Nursing: Concepts of Practice*, 1st, 2nd, 3rd, 4th 5th and 6th edns. London: Mosby.

Raudonis, B.M. and Gayle, J.A. (1997) Theory-based nursing practice. *Journal of Advanced Nursing* 26: 138–145.

Rawnsley, M.M. (1999) Response to Fawcett's 'The State of Nursing Science'. *Nursing Science Quarterly* 12(4): 315–318.

Riegel, B., Tomason, T. Carlson, B. and Gocka, L. (1996) Are nurses still practicing coronary precautions? A national survey of nursing care of acute myocardial infarction patients. *American Journal of Critical Care* 5: 91–98.

Riley, J.P., Bullock, I., West, S. and Shuldham, C. (2003) Practical application of educational rhetoric: a pathway to expert cardiac nurse practice? *European Journal of Cardiovascular Nursing* 2: 283–290.

Robinson, J. (1993) Problems with paradigms in a caring profession. In: Kitson, A. (ed) *Nursing: Art and Science*. London: Chapman Hall.

Roper, N., Logan, W.W. and Tierney, A.J. (1980, 1985, 1990,1996) *The Elements of Nursing: A Model for Nursing Based on a Model for Living*, 1st, 2nd, 3rd and 4th edns., London: Churchill Livingstone.

Roper, N., Logan, W.W. and Tierney, A.J. (2001) *The Roper Logan Tierney Model of Nursing Based on Activities of Living*. London: Churchill Livingstone.

Shamsudin, N. (2002) Can the Newman Systems Model be adapted to the Malaysian nursing context? *International Journal of Nursing Practice* 8: 99–105.

Spearman, S.A., Duldt, B.W. and Brown, S. (1993) Research testing theory: a selective review of Orem's self-care theory, 1986–1991. *Journal of Advanced Nursing* 18: 1626–1631.

Stewart, S. (2002) Cardiovascular nursing at the crossroads: are we demanding the highest academic standards? *European Journal of Cardiovascular Nursing* 1: 165–166.

Strange, F. (2001) The persistence of ritual in nursing practice. *Clinical Effectiveness in Nursing* 5(4): 177–183.

Sutcliffe, L. (1994) Philosophy and models in critical care nursing. *Intensive and Critical Care Nursing* 10: 212–221.

Taylor, S.G., Geden, E., Issaramalai, S. and Wongvatunyu, S. (2000) Orem's Self-Care Deficit Nursing Theory: its philosophic foundation and the state of the science. *Nursing Science Quarterly* 13(2): 104–108.

Thompson, D. (2002) Nurse-directed services: how can they be made more effective? *European Journal of Cardiovascular Nursing* 1: 7–10.

Tierney, A.J. (1998) 'Nursing models extant or extinct? *Journal of Advanced Nursing* 8(1): 77–85.

Timmins, F. (2002) Critical care nursing in the 21st century. *Intensive and Critical Care Nursing* 18: 118–127.

Timpson, J. (1996) Nursing theory: everything the artist spits is art? *Journal of Advanced Nursing* 23: 1030–1036.

Toulmin, S. (1972) *Human Understanding: The Collective Use and Evolution of Concepts, Princeton*. New Jersey: Princeton University Press.

Treacy, P. and Hyde, A. (1999) *Nursing Research Design and Practice*. Dublin: University College Dublin Press.

Wood, A.F. and Alligood, M.R. (2002) Nursing: normal science for nursing practice. In: Alligood, M.R. and Marriner-Tomey, A. (eds) *Nursing Theory Utilisation & Application*. London: Mosby.

Chapter 2

Planning nursing care

Key points
• Use of Orem's (2001) self-care deficit theory of nursing is suggested in coronary care settings.
• Planning nursing care using Orem's (2001) self-care framework requires investigation of the patient's universal, developmental and health deviation self-care deficits.
• Implementation of nursing care using Orem's (2001) self-care framework requires a mixture of actions unique to nursing and technological interventions.
• Critical pathways are gaining increasing popularity in coronary care settings in the UK and are suggested adjuncts to nursing practice.

Self-care deficit nursing theory in coronary care

Orem's (2001) self-care deficit nursing theory (SCDNT) is widely used and accepted by nurses (Taylor 2002) and is one of the most frequently used nursing theories in practice (Alligood and Marriner-Tomey 2002). It is also used in nursing cardiac patients (Williams and Ramos 1993, Jaarsma et al. 1998, Fawcett 1999, Jaarsma 1999).

Although the SCDNT is primarily a theory of nursing, Fawcett (1995) noted that its concepts and propositions can also be used at a practical (conceptual model) level, and therefore as a framework to guide specific nursing actions. Indeed, Orem graphically represented the relationship between elements within the SCDNT as a conceptual framework (2001: 492).

Some confusion arises with regard to terminology when considering its use in practice. Fawcett (1995) referred to 'Orem's self-care *framework*', however, commented upon its widespread use as a *conceptual model*. Orem (2001) referred to a '*conceptual framework*' and Pearson et al. (2001) in discussion and practical application of this theory referred to it as a '*self-care model*'. Orem's (2001) framework for directing nursing actions will be referred to as a *conceptual model* for the purpose of discussion in this book.

Fawcett's (1995) work is helpful for nurses in coronary care considering use of this model, as she critically appraised Orem's earlier work. The categories chosen by Fawcett (1995) for analysis (explication of origins, comprehensiveness of content, logical congruence, generation of theory and credibility) represent a comprehensive analysis of the model and comply with many of the categories in the evaluative framework discussed in Chapter 1 (Cormack and Reynolds 1992).

The analysis indicated that Orem's 'self-care framework' (conceptual model) and the 'self care deficit nursing theory' (Orem, 1990, 1991) represent a substantial contribution to nursing knowledge through the provision of an explicit and specific focus for nursing actions that is different from that of other healthcare professions. 'Orem has fulfilled her goal of identifying the domain and boundaries of nursing as a science and an art' (Fawcett 1995: 339).

This is a useful observation. Cormack and Reynolds (1992) suggest that a conceptual model should 'outline an approach that is specific to nurses and nursing' and this model certainly fulfils these criteria. At a time when the boundaries of nursing practice, particularly in coronary care are becoming blurred with extension and advancement of nursing roles, it is essential that as nurses, we retain a focus on what it is that nurses do and should do. This could also pacify those who sense the demise of modern nursing (Fawcett 1999), by clearly defining nursing roles within practice settings. Orem (2001) outlines the nurse's unique function to an even greater extent.

Orem's seminal texts on the topic (1971, 1980, 1985, 1995) have undergone much evolution and development over the years. The most recent edition in 2001 contains new content that examines nursing in a general context. Orem outlines the nursing contribution to practice. This theme is developed as the SCDNT – a general theory that outlines what nursing is and should be. Thus it is a general, rather than a specific guide to practice.

A brief description of the SCDNT will be useful to aid understanding. The underlying assumptions of the theory include:

- individuals require continuous personal and environmental input in order to function effectively
- human *agency* (the ability to act deliberately), involves self-care and care of others that is based upon needs
- mature humans can experience limitations on this (self-care and care of others)
- this agency develops over time, and enables oneself or others to provide inputs to ensure effective functioning.

The SCDNT incorporates three intertwining theories (Orem 2001).

- Theory of self-care
- Theory of self-care deficit
- Theory of nursing systems

The theory of self-care was a cornerstone in the development of the SCDNT. Orem defined self-care as 'a human regulatory function that individuals with deliberation perform for themselves or have performed for them (dependent-care) to supply and maintain a supply of materials and conditions to maintain life...' (2001: 143). Self-care, she suggests, must be *learned* and performed deliberately. This theory assumes that all mature and maturing persons develop and use skills to enable them to take care of themselves and their dependants.

The theory of self-care deficit outlines why individuals require nursing care.

> Requirements of persons for nursing are associated with the subjectivity of
> mature and maturing persons to health-derived or healthcare-related action
> limitations associated with their own or their dependants' health states that
> render them completely or partially unable to know existent and emerging
> requisites for regularity care for themselves or their dependents . . .
>
> (Orem 2001: 146)

Nursing care is required for individuals when their needs for care exceed their
own ability to meet these needs. Nursing is required when an individual's self-care
abilities are less than, or predicted to become less than, those required for meeting a
known self-care demand. This is known as 'a deficit relationship'. A self-care deficit
may be permanent or transitory.

The theory of nursing systems is the unifying theory and includes all the essential
elements. It subsumes the theory of self-care deficit and the theory of self-care. This
theory proposes that nursing is a human action – formed (designed and produced)
by nurses through the exercise of their nursing agency for people with health-derived
or health-associated limitations in self-care or dependent-care. Nursing agency
includes concepts of deliberate action.

SCDNT is useful to nurses in coronary care. Using this theory to understand and
describe the nursing situation can have a direct impact on practice. A nurse's personal theory or framework affects their view of the patient and the healthcare situation. If they, for example, view the patient as a condition, demonstrated by the old
adage of 'the MI in bed four', they may see their role as primarily assisting cure and
providing care. This may manifest itself in a nursing role concerned with providing
pharmacological interventions, assisting with and preparing for invasive techniques
and providing (perhaps routine) physical care (for example assisting with personal
hygiene and mobility needs). Operating from this frame of reference leads to the
possibility of the patient being viewed as the dependent receiver of hospital care and
can lead to individual disempowerment.

The SCDNT on the other hand empowers patients. Patients presenting to the coronary care unit are understood and acknowledged as being independent in their life
prior to admission (either through caring for themselves (self-care) or care by others
(dependent-care)). This understanding facilitates respect for patients and individualised care. An event that disrupts this independence, resulting in a self-care deficit
prompts this patient's presentation to the hospital. Already we can see that using this
framework alters our thinking about patients. It moves us away from the medical
model of care. Nursing serves to address, in a personable way, the limitations imposed
on the patient's self-care, due to their condition. Rather than initiating a prescribed list
of treatment interventions in a routine way, the nurse determines the nature and
amount of self-care requisite of each individual and the nature of technological interventions and adjunct nursing care required to support these. This is a complex
process, highlighting the unique skills of the nurse who engages with the patient (and
family) to assess the therapeutic self-care demand of each individual.

The term therapeutic self-care demand relates to the 'amount and kind of self-
care that persons should have' (Orem 2001) and is fundamental to the SCDNT. It
refers to courses of action or care measures that must be performed to fulfil the
goals of self-care requisites of individuals (Orem 2001). The concept must be

---

Box 2.1 Universal self-care requisites

1. Maintenance of a sufficient intake of air
2. Maintenance of a sufficient intake of water
3. Maintenance of a sufficient intake of food
4. Provision of care associated with elimination processes and excrements
5. Maintenance of balance between activity and rest
6. Maintenance of balance between solitude and social interaction
7. Prevention of hazards to human life, human functioning, and human wellbeing
8. Promotion of human functioning and development within social groups in accordance with human potential, known human limitations and the human desire to be normal

Adapted from Orem, D.E. (2001) *Nursing: Concepts of Practice* (6th edn). London: Mosby.

---

constructed by nurses in practice situations through an assessment and decision-making process to determine the nature and amount of self-care requisite (see above) and the nature of technological interventions and adjunct nursing care required to support these (Orem 2001). Orem (2001: 224) suggested that nurses must be 'dynamic in their knowing and be proficient in the use of developed intellectual and perceptual skills to engage in the complex process of calculating persons' therapeutic self-care demands'. The nurse assesses therapeutic self-care demand through analysis of therapeutic self-care requisites in three distinct domains: universal, developmental and health deviation.

Universal self-care requisites are universally required goals that are met through self-care or dependent-care. Eight self-care requisites common to all were identified by Orem (2001) and are displayed in Box 2.1.

These eight requisites represent actions that result in conditions that maintain human functioning, and support human development. When effectively provided, self-care or dependent-care, based on the universal self-care requisites, promotes health and wellbeing. General sets of actions for meeting the eight requisites have been outlined by Orem (2001: 227). Meeting the universal self-care requisites through self-care or dependent-care is an integral component of the daily living of individuals and groups.

Developmental self-care requisites were initially a component of universal self-care requisites, but Orem (2001) reports that they have been separated out to emphasise their importance. She states that the identification and expression of these requisites is difficult. They are concerned with all aspects of human development, which are defined as flexible, dynamic processes, events and occurrences, and functioning that occur in each individual. These requisites promote processes for life and maturation and prevent conditions deleterious to maturation or those that mitigate those effects (Orem 2001). Three sets of developmental requisites, provision of conditions that promote development, engagement in self-development and interferences with development have been outlined by Orem (2001).

Conditions that promote development are requisites met by dependent-care agents in the early stages of life. These include the provision of physical and emotional conditions and experiences that foster physical and emotional development.

Engagement in self-development, that emerges later in life, requires deliberate involvement of self in the process.

Interferences with development suggest that there is a need to provide conditions and promote behaviours that will prevent or overcome the occurrence of deleterious effects on development. Such effects include poor health.

Health deviation self-care requisites are self-care requisites for individuals who are ill or injured, who have specific forms of pathological conditions or disorders, including defects and disabilities, and who are undergoing medical treatment. The characteristics of health deviation as conditions extending over time determine the kinds of care demands that individuals experience as they live with the effects of pathological conditions through their duration (Orem 2001). When health status changes resulting in total or almost total dependence upon others to sustain life or wellbeing, the individual moves from the position of self-care agent to that of receiver of care. Seeking and participating in medical care for health deviation are self-care actions.

Although not explicitly stated in the model, the nursing process underpins the operation of the model in practice. This information is transferred to a care plan. The first stage for nurses when using this model is *assessment*. This 'calculation and design' of the therapeutic self-care demand requires an 'investigative process' (Orem 2001: 247). The three domains of therapeutic self-care discussed above specify a wide range of requisites pertinent to the coronary care situation and provide for comprehensive and holistic planning of patient care. Many cardiac conditions are due to a physiological condition that affects universal self-care requisites and health deviation self-care demand. It addition, the potentially serious or life-threatening nature of many conditions treated in coronary care units prompt emotional reactions in patients, which may be identified as developmental requisites. This latter aspect of coronary care nursing is quite underdeveloped and use of this model facilitates nursing action in this area.

Planning describes and prescribes the amount of care that an individual requires. It involves outlining the actions (related to human functioning and development) that the individual should perform or have performed by another within a specific timeframe. In practice, this requires the identification (and documentation) of self-care requisites and the processes for meeting these, i.e. the identification of conditions that enable or obstruct the individual's ability to meet the requisite and outlining technologies, methods and actions that will meet the requisites.

Intervention involves nursing systems, a series of deliberate (collaborative with patient) practical actions to meet patients' therapeutic self-care demands and to protect and promote patients' self-care agency (ability to meet their own needs) (Orem 2001). Within this nursing system, nursing care can be described and implemented on a continuum ranging from wholly compensatory (doing for the patient), partly compensatory (helping the patient to do for him or herself) or supportive-educative (helping the patient learn to do for him or herself).

Orem (2001) views nurses very much in a helping role. She defined nursing systems as 'helping systems', whereby the nurse's role involves several identified methods of helping such as (Orem 2001: 349):

- acting for or doing for another
- guiding and directing

- providing physical or psychological support
- providing and maintaining an environment that supports personal development
- teaching.

In summary, using SCDNT to guide nursing practice in coronary care provides nurses with an understanding that nursing action is required for individuals when their needs (self-care requisites) exceed their own ability to meet these needs resulting in a self-care deficit. Using this conceptual model in coronary care practice involves performing and documenting an assessment, whereby the patient's level of therapeutic healthcare demand is estimated through examination of the universal, health deviation and developmental requisites.

Plan of care is concerned with outlining of planned provision of helping methods and wholly compensatory/partially compensatory/supportive-educative nursing care, together with an outline of required technologies to effectively meet the patient's requisites. Evaluation is the final stage where the nurse establishes whether (or to what extent) nursing systems achieved goals of care.

Applying conceptual models in coronary care nursing

Although conceptual models guide nursing actions in a general sense, the specifics of formulating individualised care plans and devising associated documents for use in particular areas such as coronary care is a notable exception from the literature. This also applies to the SCDNT model. While there are some examples in texts such as Aggleton and Chambers (2000), few specifically relate to the coronary care setting. In addition, those that do exist in the literature to date refer to earlier editions of the model (Orem 1971, 1980, 1985, 1995) and not to the most recent version (2001).

One way of guiding coronary care practice, therefore is by examining the work of other writers who have described the use and application of this conceptual model to cardiac patients and/or critical care. This provides understanding regarding the extent to which the model may be suitable for the coronary care setting.

Some guidelines are there in the literature on specific use of Orem's conceptual model with cardiac patients, with some developmental work emerging on heart failure patients (Jaarsma et al. 1998, Jaarsma 1999) and patients with a mitral valve prolapse (Williams and Ramos 1993) in addition to one case study of a patient following complicated myocardial infarction (Fawcett et al. 1992).

Fawcett (a seminal author in conceptual model analysis) and her colleagues in 1992 outlined six case studies using Orem's conceptual model including one describing the care of a patient who suffered a myocardial infarction, subsequent ventricular fibrillation cardiac arrest, underwent percutaneous transluminal angioplasty (PTCA) and required an automatic implantable defibrillator (AICD).

Fawcett et al. (1992) claimed that the fit between this patient and Orem's self-care framework was 'perfect'. In the initial phase, the patient experienced health-related self-care requisites due to chest pain. The associated symptoms created a therapeutic self-care demand that exceeded his self-care agency and creating a self-care deficit that required him to seek medical and nursing care (Fawcett et al. 1992). During the cardiac arrest, and in the period immediately after this, the nurses delivered complete care – deemed wholly compensatory in Orem's model.

During the patient's various phases of recovery he was able to participate more in his care and the nursing care was only partially compensatory (Fawcett et al. 1992). Following the insertion of the AICD the supportive-educative system was used to assist the patient with learning how to live with the device. Each nursing care system was delivered with an ultimate aim of patient self-care. This patient progressed from wholly compensatory through the partially compensatory to the supportive-educative nursing system as his related self-care requisites decreased. Finally, his therapeutic self-care demand was balanced by enhanced self-care agency and the self-care deficits were no longer evident (Fawcett et al. 1992).

This case study clearly illustrates the ability of the SCDNT to transform a patient from dependent recipient to active participant. Outlining the nursing care required on a progressive continuum from wholly compensatory to supportive-educative empowered the patient towards independence and restored self-care.

Jaarsma (1999) examined the supportive-educative aspect of the nursing action to illustrate how Orem's (1995) SCDNT aided the development of an education programme for patients with heart failure. By applying the information in the literature, standard nursing care plans and nurse interviews to the situation of a patient with heart failure, Jaarsma concluded that requisites existed in each of the eight universal self-care requisites because of heart failure and its treatment. Jaarsma therefore focused education on this area.

Williams and Ramos (1993) described the therapeutic self-care demands of people with symptomatic mitral valve prolapse (MVP): 'Extant medical research and copious clinical nursing experience led researchers to the belief that people with symptomatic MVP had nursing care needs that could be addressed successfully through the use of Orem's framework'. Their study involved reviewing medical records and patient interviews. The findings revealed that patients expressed needs in all six categories of health deviation self-care requisites (Box 2.2). The predominant concerns included perceived need for (i) acceptance by others (including healthcare personnel) of

---

Box 2.2 Health deviation self-care requisites of patients with MVP identified by Williams and Ramos (1993)

- Seeking and securing appropriate medical assistance
- Being aware of and attending to the effects and results of pathological conditions and states
- Effectively carrying out medically prescribed measures
- Being aware of and attending to or regulating the discomforting or deleterious effects of medical care measures
- Modifying the self-concept in accepting oneself as being in a particular state of health and in need of special forms of healthcare
- Learning to live with the effects of health state and treatment in a lifestyle that promotes continued personal development

Adapted from Williams, S. and Ramos, M.C. (1993) Mitral valve prolapse and its effects: a programme of inquiry within Orem's Self-Care Deficit Theory of nursing. *Journal of Advanced Nursing* 18: 742–751.

subjective discomfort, (ii) an understanding of the condition and (iii) help with symptom management and lifestyle adjustment.

Williams and Ramos (1993) also surveyed 34 nurses and outlined methods of nursing assistance that were commonly used. This revealed frequent use of helping actions such as:

- teaching (70%)
- guiding and directing (53%)
- acting for or doing for another (41%)
- providing physical or psychological support (53%).

One item that concerns us as nurses is whether using a conceptual model has an overall impact on patient care. Few studies have examined outcomes with regard to conceptual model use. One study (Aish and Isenberg 1996) investigated the effects of nursing care based on Orem's (1985, 1991) SCDNT on nutritional self-care of 104 patients who had suffered a myocardial infarction for the first time.

Nutritional self-care was measured using a diet record and a questionnaire. An experimental group received nursing nutritional intervention based on Orem's (1991) recommendations over a 6-week period. The control group received usual care. The findings revealed that the nursing intervention was effective in supporting the necessary dietary changes.

From the papers discussed above, Orem's (2001) SCDNT emerges as a suitable framework to guide nursing practice in coronary care.

Critical pathways

The perceived complexity of conceptual model use, scepticism and problems with use in practice, such as time-consuming documentation, have led many coronary care nurses in the UK to embrace alternatives. Care pathways are becoming an increasingly popular method of planning nursing care in the UK. Their use has also been reported in Australia (Gibson and Heartfield 1996). The dissatisfaction noted by Mason with conceptual-model-based care plan use prompted him to suggest that 'a reinvention of the nursing care plan is needed, without the constraint of a nursing model as the necessary foundation' (1999: 387).

Mason (1999) indicated that there were benefits with the use of 'alternative plans' such as care pathways, suggesting that conceptual model use is not essential. However, Mason highlights that use of pathways may erode conceptual models from nursing practice settings in the UK. This factor needs to be considered. Indeed when Stead and Huckle (1997) described the development and introduction of integrated cardiology care pathways at St Mary's Hospital, London, UK (myocardial infarction, angina, PTCA, stent and pacemaker insertion, radio frequency ablation), concerns emerged such as that they would replace individualised care, remove autonomy by dictating care, would replace the nursing process and potentially eliminate conceptual nursing models of care. However, Stead and Huckle reported that when the scheme was introduced the staff's response was favourable and 'immense' benefits were conferred upon interdisciplinary communication and quality, practice and costs.

While care pathways have potential benefits for nursing practice, their use also needs careful scrutiny to ensure that nursing practice is based on the *best* evidence and not the latest evidence. It is also important that nursing retains its endeavours to develop a strong theoretical foundation, as this is more likely to contribute to the generation of knowledge in practice as opposed to the use of plans in isolation.

It appears from the literature that conceptual model use has become synonymous with documentation and care planning. From a nurse's perspective these are the day-to-day concerns related to the delivery of conceptual-model-based nursing care. However the use of conceptual models should represent a paradigm shift in nurses' thinking and practice. They serve to move away from ritual and tradition long associated with nursing to thoughtful planned care. They intend to outline a delivery of care that is distinctly nursing and quite different from that of other health professionals. They also aim to be patient centred; goals of nursing are usually patient-focused and cater for patients' needs and priorities from social, psychological and emotional perspectives.

To some extent the use of care pathways represent a retrograde step in nursing practice. They provide standardised care packages focusing on cost savings and efficiency at the expense of the individual. Individualised nursing care has been the hallmark of contemporary nursing. While the practice may be retained, the underlying philosophy of pathways is reductionistic, which is the antithesis of modern nursing.

Care pathways, originally used in the USA, have become increasingly popular in the UK, although not necessarily in other parts of Europe. This is due in part to the economic and political climates of these two nations. The private healthcare corporations in the USA drive the need for cost-effective care. Cost containment is also an issue in the UK, although for different reasons linked with the economy and health budget synonymous with the political agendas of the 1980s and 1990s (Jones and Tucker 2000). The use of care pathways in the UK is strongly associated with the current nationally driven quality initiatives and policies of standard setting. It is also related to the ease with which these tools can facilitate audit and quality assurance (Riley 1998).

While many academics remain sceptical, many practising nurses are tired of 'outdated' practices and are of the opinion that 'this level of traditional nursing practice is at an unacceptable standard' (Herring 1999). For Herring (1999) pathways are an obvious alternative and pathways have replaced traditional nursing care plans in many areas. Walsh (1998) argues that pathways and the traditional process are not competitors; they are two aspects of the same approach to care – although current evidence suggests that they are for the most part used independently of conceptual models of nursing.

While theory and conceptual model development could be said to emanate from the professional and academic development of the nursing profession, care pathways have had a different conception. Many terms are used to describe care pathways, often interchangeable, although there are subtle differences in practical application (Johnson 1997a: 4). The term 'care pathway' is often used as a generic term to cover all the different applications of pathways including integrated care pathways, clinical pathways, anticipated recovery pathways and critical pathways.

In the UK, rather than emphasising the aim of controlling costs, care pathways are seen as a tool to implement clinical governance that can improve the quality of care and ensure that clinical care is based on the latest evidence and research. The National Pathways Association (NPA) outlines the function of a care pathway as follows: 'a care pathway determines locally agreed, multi-disciplinary practice based on guidelines and evidence where available, for a specific patient or client group. It forms all or part of the clinical record, documents the care given and facilitates the evaluation of outcomes' (Riley 1998).

In the UK, the Department of Health endorses the use of care pathways. The White Paper, *The New NHS: Modern and Dependable* outlined updated arrangements for commissioning services through the introduction of long-term service agreements (LTSAs) (Department of Health 1998a,b). A shared view of outcomes of care was highlighted, as being crucial to these agreements and pathways of care were a suggested tool, not only to aid common understanding of outcomes but also to ensure effective use of resources and setting efficiency targets. It was envisaged that the LTSAs would eventually be totally based on pathways of care for specific conditions, rather than other elements of the National Health Service (NHS) facilities.

Riley (1998) brought to our attention the development of the NPA in the UK. This aimed to provide information for organisations developing pathways. The association carried out a survey of members (n = 94) in 1997 to establish pathway usage. The survey revealed that pathways were most popular among NHS trust hospitals, although their use was also reported in private facilities. Orthopaedic surgery was the most frequently cited speciality that used pathways and 28 hospitals reported using pathways in cardiology or cardiothoracic surgery. Multi-disciplinary documentation was present in 92% of cases. They were also used as all or part of clinical patient records (92%), incorporated into guidelines (92%) and incorporated into quality standards of care (85%). Pathways were useful in setting and implementing standards of care, improving quality care, improving intraprofessional communication, and promoting evidence-based practice. However, very few respondents agreed that pathways assisted in cost control (37%) with 30% reporting their use to be of no use or slightly useful in controlling costs. The most important aspect of successful implementation was clinical ownership/amenability to change.

Similar findings were revealed by De Luc (2000) who explored the views of seven staff members to the use of care pathways for breast care using critical incident technique. Positive aspects of pathway use were revealed as aiding the setting and monitoring of standards, prompting action, improving continuity and improving multi-disciplinary communication. Negative comments included references to the lack of ownership and change in clinical care and concern around pathway documentation.

The views of five midwives were also elicited in a similar fashion in the same study. Favourable comments related to improvements in clinical care and making the care more patient-focused. All eight unfavourable comments concerned pathway documentation.

Care pathways have been embraced by practising general nurses in the UK across a wide range of specialities. Their simplistic nature and ease of understanding contribute to this. In addition, ensuring that patients receive standardised, documented care, easily monitored for variations is reassuring to the profession that has intrinsic high standards. The multi-disciplinary nature of many of the pathways is also attractive, fosters good relations and improves work satisfaction.

This wide range of interest in care pathways is reflected in other occupational groups such as doctors. A number of textbooks outline the nature and process of care pathways in both nursing and medicine and there is some published empirical evidence in anecdotal and review pieces as well as management texts supporting their use. In general, they appear to be a useful adjunct to care delivery. There is also a journal dedicated to pathways, *Journal of Integrated Care Pathways*, a publication with an international outlook and a forum for exploring a wide range of issues relating to care pathway use. An integrated care pathway conference is held every year in the UK. These indicate the level of enthusiasm and commitment in the UK with regard to care pathway use.

This enthusiasm is also reflected in the NHS National electronic Library for Protocols and Care Pathways (NeLPCP) (NHS 2003a), a component of the National electronic Library for Health (NeLH) (NHS 2003b). The website was launched in 2001 and provides a Care Pathways Database containing more than 2000 entries from more than 200 NHS organisations indicating the high level of commitment to care pathways that exists in practice. The NPA (2003) also provides a network for professionals interested in sharing ideas and promoting care pathway usage. It acts as a national resource on pathways and facilitates research into care pathways.

One area where care pathways may gain credence over conceptuals-model-based care is in relation to outcome. While there is a dearth of evidence supporting the overall benefits of conceptual-model-based care on patient outcome, there is empirical evidence suggesting that pathway use has a beneficial effect on length of patient stay and reduction in complications. As improving patient outcome is a major goal of healthcare, these facts inspire confidence in their use.

Despite the popularity of care pathways, Johnson (1997b) and De Luc (2000) stated that there is little empirical evidence to support their use in the UK and recommend immediate evaluation of effectiveness. 'Most sites pilot their use based on anecdotal success stories from other pathway user sites. As a National Health Service we are overdue in commissioning valid research to comprehensively evaluate the use of pathways' (Johnson 1997b: 4).

A Cochrane systematic review (Kwan and Sandercock 1999) of the use of care pathways for stroke patients revealed conflicting reports. The review aimed to assess the effects of care pathways, as compared with standard medical care, among patients with acute stroke admitted to hospital. Three randomised controlled trials (n = 340) were identified and seven non-randomised (n = 1673) comparing the use of care pathway with standard care. No differences were found between care pathway groups and control groups regarding outcomes related to death, dependency, or discharge destination.

Kwan and Sandercock (1999) observed that evidence from mostly non-randomised studies suggests that patients managed using a care pathway are less likely to suffer a urinary tract infection and their re-admission rate is lower. On the other hand evidence from randomised trials suggests that patient satisfaction and quality of life may actually be lower in the care pathway groups. They concluded that the use of care pathways to manage stroke patients in hospital might be associated with both positive and negative effects on the process of care and clinical outcomes.

Although care pathway terminology is used interchangeably, *critical* pathways, which are popular in critical care areas, denote pathways that have been developed for specific conditions and operate for the duration of the condition and not necessarily the duration of the patient stay. Critical pathways represent the organisation's effort to promote consistent clinical outcomes and control costs. Wall and Proyect (1998) point out that there are a variety of different interpretations of the term 'critical pathway', and little consensus exists regarding its definition. They define clinical pathway as that which outlines every element of care required daily for the entire duration of an episode, regardless of its impact on outcomes, whereas critical pathway is defined an outline of a small number of essential elements in a treatment regimen which have proven impact on clinical or financial outcomes of care.

Critical pathways have been suggested for use in coronary care. Cannon and O'Gara (2001), for example, outlined critical pathways for use in many acute clinical areas in their seminal text. This included detailed critical pathway description for 'the chest pain patient at low risk', 'unstable angina' and 'congestive heart failure'.

A recent review of the literature revealed that critical pathways are effective in enhancing outcomes of patient care (Renholm et al. 2002). In this review several patient care outcomes were positively affected in the studies examined including patient satisfaction, continuity of care, continuity of information, length of hospital stay, reduction in costs. Several studies have examined the effect of critical pathways on patient outcome, namely, reduction in costs including length of hospital stay and reduction in complications.

Reduction in costs including length of hospital stay

In the USA, Wammack and Mabrey (1999) examined cost-effectiveness of critical pathways: complications, re-admission rate, morbidity/mortality figures, and function scores of two groups of patients undergoing total hip and knee arthroplasties who attended before and after the implementation of critical pathways at the hospital. Their findings revealed that the length of stay was reduced by 57% for knee patients and by 46% for hip patients. Hospital costs were reduced by 11% for all knees and 38% for hips, although this was not statistically significant.

In another orthopaedic setting in the USA, Ireson (1997) found a decrease in hospitalisation time of 1.45 days with the use of critical pathways. The mean charge for the critical pathway group was 6% less than for the care plan group, but the difference was not statistically significant.

Reduction in complications

While Wammack and Mabrey (1999) revealed overall benefits of cost, use of critical pathways for orthopaedic patients had little overall benefit in patient outcome, when compared with usual care. While complications were reduced, the results were not significant. In addition, there was no statistically significant difference between pre- and post-operative knee or hip outcome scores.

Ireson (1997) also compared outcomes in patients having total knee or hip replacements to examine whether or not differences emerged between discharge outcomes when critical pathways were used instead of the traditional process of nursing care plans. A total of 128 patients were included in the study, split evenly into the control and experimental groups. The variables included clinical quality, length of hospital stay, and financial outcomes. A quasi-experimental design with repeated measures was used to compare patient outcomes using a critical pathway with outcomes using a hospital's standardised care plan. The findings revealed that patients cared for with a critical pathway achieved better outcomes on the day before discharge.

Gibson and Heartfield (1996) noted that while many authors identify and outline the function of critical pathways, their impact on health personnel, settings and patients is rarely addressed. Furthermore, they suggest that 'authors writing about critical pathways rarely take a critical perspective'. They critically analysed critical pathways under the heading of 'language text and content' and 'bureaucratic control of nursing knowledge'. Gibb and Banfield (1996) are critical of the nursing passivity with regard to critical pathway use. They note that there is almost universal 'collective uncritical acceptance' of their value with little thought given to critical evaluation of their potential.

The authors cited above consider critical pathway use to conflict with the inherent values and current discourse within nursing. They note that there is little space for writing comments on critical pathway documentation, so valuable patient descriptors are omitted. Individualised holistic care is abandoned and the complexity of nursing care is reduced to a 'tick'. Upon examination of critical pathways they suggest there is an obvious over-reliance on physical aspects of care and medical interventions resulting in 'constructions of the patient as an object and a commodified body'. The patient's role becomes passive 'a silent, passive object; a body subjected to healthcare interventions and defined in terms of the standard or deviation from the standard'. These observations are concerning given nursing's efforts to detach itself from the medical model of care in favour of more inclusive psychosocial models. Gibson and Heartfield (1996) questioned the value of supposed collaborative care, suggesting that this actually disempowered nurses. Furthermore, they questioned whether it is realistic or possible to develop tools that can potentially reflect the unique approach of more than one discipline.

Holt et al. (1996) provide a summary of key national activities in the development and implementation of critical pathways in New South Wales. Data were collected by means of structured interview and included 138 individuals from 61 organisations. The findings revealed that the term critical pathway was well understood as 'a documented plan of expected clinical management where the critical treatments and interventions are identified and sequenced along a timeline' (Holt et al. 1996). Pathways were used exclusively within hospitals and their use did not normally extend beyond discharge. They were usually developed for high-volume procedures (usually surgical interventions) and reflected consensus-based care rather than care based on evidence.

Scott (2002: 565) suggested that the many technological and medical advances in cardiac practice in recent years means that 'pre-existing models of nursing may not offer the flexibility to address the requirements of current cardiac practice'. She states that the ability of critical pathways for care planning emerges in the literature but cautions that 'it still remains important to explore the utility and effectiveness of this new export from the United States in fully addressing ... management and clinic issues before adopting the process' (2002: 565). She defines the critical pathway as 'the tool of managed care which facilitates delivery and audit of patient care' (2002: 566).

'It is a blank template on which the multi-disciplinary team describe standardised patterns of care and key interventions of all disciplines which need to be carried out sequentially for the patient's specific condition' (2002: 556). In her research study critical pathways were introduced solely as a quality initiative and not for cost-effectiveness, although this was a perceived benefit. She outlined crucial steps in the development and implementation of critical pathways: building the multi-disciplinary team, developing a common philosophy of care, making the implicit explicit, designing the critical pathway and use in practice. She also suggests that the pathway should be 'scrutinised and ratified by senior nurses and consultants before use in practice' (2002: 576).

Potential pitfalls with the use of critical pathways were identified by Polanczyk and Lee (2001) including the inherent difficulty with assessment of their effectiveness as evidenced by empirical studies due to methodological limitations such as lack of randomised controls. Polanczyk and Lee (2001) suggest that positive findings reported in the literature must be viewed with caution due to the possibility of reporter bias leading to over-representation of positive studies in the literature.

Gibson and Heartfield (1996) and Scott (2002) advocate a cautious and critical approach to adoption of critical pathways in nursing practice. This supports McSherry et al.'s (2002) view that nurses should be critical practitioners: 'nurses are employed as experts – they are paid to practise on the basis that what they do is well-judged, appropriate and based on an informed appraisal of alternatives'. Examining the knowledge base that informs practice is a crucial element of critical practice (Brechin 2000) and critical appraisal of pathways rather than passive adoption is advised.

Specific critical appraisal guidelines for critical pathway use have not been identified in the literature, however, Wall and Proyect (1998: ix) outlined a guide for implementing and developing critical pathways. Strategies for critical pathway development within the coronary care unit are described below.

Developing care pathways

Wall and Proyect (1998: ix) suggest that critical pathways should either be developed or modified locally to suit particular needs of the specific patient group, rather than using an available pathway. They outline a five-step process for developing and implementing critical pathways, known as the 'Quality Team Associates (QTA) Critical Pathway Model' (1998: 1).

Critical pathways represent an organisation's effort to promote consistent clinical outcomes and control costs. They have been tried in a multitude of healthcare settings and have in some areas 'become a way of life for clinicians' (Wall and Proyect 1998: 3). As mentioned above there are a variety of different interpretations of the term 'critical pathway', and little consensus regarding its definition. Several other terms are used interchangeably: clinical pathways, care paths, anticipated recovery paths. However, Wall and Proyect (1998) point out that while many view these terms as synonymous, others contend that there are important distinctions between them.

Wall and Proyect suggest that prior to embarking on a project to develop and implement pathways, a standard term for the pathway must be clearly outlined and understood. This can be done by establishing what terminology is most widely accepted in the area and also by examining existing definitions.

Despite the variation in approaches to critical pathways, Wall and Proyect (1998) suggest that commonalities exist. All critical pathways are designed for a specific patient population, they represent consensus among healthcare providers, identify patient outcomes and are the result of careful consideration and systematic validation. Their rationale for the development and implementation of critical pathways includes managing limited financial resources, implementing changes in the patient care delivery process and making efficient use of organisational resources.

Wall and Proyect (1998) outline five steps for the development and implementation of the QTA Critical Pathway Model. First, identify the target population and pathway boundaries. This may be done by developing selection criteria, reviewing available data, selecting patient population and defining pathway boundaries. Secondly, develop the critical pathway. This involves establishing critical pathway goals, reviewing the literature, identify how goals may be met, collect internal practice data, negotiate critical pathway elements, obtain agreement. Thirdly, the pathway is implemented. This entails establishing an implementation schedule, assigning responsibilities, developing support tools and providing education. Implementation involves selecting locations for implementation, preparing documentation, preparing guidelines for administration, and conducting a pilot test. Following implementation, in the fourth step the results are measured by collecting pathway information and analysing data. Finally, the pathway results are utilised to reinforce desired performance, identify key areas for revision and updating and to implement required revisions to the pathway. Participation and communication are crucial to pathway development (Wall and Proyect 1998).

Inatavicius and Hausmann (1995) have also outlined methods for development and implementation of pathways. They identified two key factors necessary for the successful implementation: support from the hospital's administration team and resources. They also suggest the appointment of a project officer to lead the development, as this commitment of dedicated staff is more likely to yield success.

Multi-disciplinary support for the project is essential and this may be facilitated through information dissemination and sharing of ideas. They also suggest that once support for the development is established, a steering group may be established to guide the project.

Inatavicius and Hausmann (1995) suggest that the selection of the pathway involves three steps: selection of the target pathway, establishment of the outcome(s) to achieve by using a pathway for the target population and determination of aspects of care to include in the pathway.

The literature has many examples of care pathways and there are many descriptions of pathways for coronary care. Stead and Huckle (1997) include an ICP (integrated care pathway) for myocardial infarction patients. Inatavicius and Hausmann (1995) outlined 33 clinical pathways for medical/surgical patients including clinical pathways for patients with uncomplicated myocardial infarction, whose expected length of hospital stay is 4 days, patients with congestive heart failure with an expected hospitalisation of 5 days. Eight pathways are included for critical care patients, including pathways for patients with complicated myocardial infarction (length of stay 6 days) and PTCA (length of stay 3 days).

Another strength of pathway use is the focus on evaluation of the process. The pathway usually contains key elements of care and treatment for a particular condition or disease. Its documentation often takes the form of a grid, indicating a timescale at the top (days or hours) and a vertical list of interventions. Deviations occurring with the use of the plan in practice are called 'variances'. Through analysis of the level and number of variances with a particular condition current practice can be monitored (Johnson 1997c). These data can then be used to update and improve clinical and practices by incorporating any new changes within the overall pathway template, thus completing the audit cycle (Kitchiner et al. 1996, Campbell et al. 1998). The pathway becomes a dynamic tool continually being refined.

The use of a critical pathway to plan nursing care, is less reliant on individual assessment than is the use of a conceptual model. The central tenet of the pathway is that standardised care is administered to the patient based on locally agreed standards. Deviations from these (variances) can be recorded, analysed and addressed at local level to improve practice.

The advocates of pathways list many benefits of their use including: greater consistency in practice; improved continuity of care; the ability to improve and monitor standards; improved clinical documentation (Kitchiner et al. 1996, Campbell et al. 1998). However, inconsistencies exist in the literature regarding improvement outcome, and there is purported to be a potential over-reporting of positive results. It is imperative, therefore, that care pathway use is integrated into practice cautiously. In the absence of firm evidence to support their use the most appropriate action is to use care pathways as an adjunct to care. Their use for audit purposes is reported throughout the literature.

Many authors have highlighted the concern regarding the depletion of conceptual model use in practice including the many nurses identified in Stead and Huckle's (1997) study. Clearly, urgent action is needed to preserve the development of the theoretical basis of nursing practice and to restore conceptual models to the practice setting with possible integration of critical pathways as appropriate. Walsh (1998: 102) cautions against 'blanket implementation' of critical pathways suggesting they are but one potential tool. Walsh (1998: 103) also recommends that the conceptual nursing model 'is not lost' and describes the potential of 'building Orem's self-care model into a CP [critical pathway] for stroke patients' (1998: 104). Clearly the future in this area is a kaleidoscope of possibility. Practising nurses need to be at the forefront of this development. The use of conceptual models has over the years served to individualise nursing care to each patient. There is concern that standardising care for conditions is a retrograde step in this notion of individualism. Indeed when Lee et al. (2002) investigated the use of a computerised care plan system in a Taiwan intensive care unit, one theme that emerged from the qualitative data pertained to the 'de-individualization of care plan' which was of great concern to the 12 nurses in question.

Summary and conclusions

A lot of work clearly needs to be done in this area to investigate methods of preserving the essence of nursing in an era of cost and quality concerns. Multi-disciplinary approaches to care are vital, however, not at the cost of holistic patient care or blurring of the boundaries of the art of nursing. More empirical evidence is required to elicit the problems that emerge with conceptual model use in practice and should aim to address these. Further evaluative research needs to be carried out to assess the effectiveness of critical pathways and potential for using this concept in conjunction with conceptual models as advocated by Walsh (1998). Coronary care nurses consider critical pathway use or development must adopt a critical stance and systematic approach to their implementation. This should include consideration of the extent to which the critical pathway can be integrated into nursing care that is directed by conceptual model use.

References

Aggleton, S.K. and Chambers, H. (2000) *Nursing Models and Nursing Practice*, 2nd edn. London: Macmillan Press.

Aish, A.E. and Isenberg, M. (1996) Effects of Orem-based nursing intervention on nutritional self-care of myocardial infarction patients. *International Journal of Nursing Studies* 33(3): 259–270.

Alligood, M.R. and Marriner-Tomey, A. (2002) (eds) *Nursing Theorists and Their Work*, 5th edn. London: Mosby.

Brechin, A. (2000) Introducing critical practice. In: Brechin, A., Brown, H. and Eby, M. (eds) *Critical Practice in Health and Social Care*. London: Sage Publications.

Campbell, H., Hotchkiss, R., Bradshaw, N. and Porteous, M. (1998) Integrated care pathways. *British Medical Journal* 316: 133–137.

Cannon, C.P. and O'Gara, P.T. (2001) (eds) *Critical Pathways in Cardiology*. Philadelphia: Lippincott Williams and Wilkins.

Cormack, D.F.S. and Reynolds, W. (1992) Criteria for evaluating the clinical and practical utility of models used by nurses. *Journal of Advanced Nursing* 17: 1472–1478.

De Luc, K. (2000) Care pathways: an evaluation of their effectiveness. *Journal of Advanced Nursing* 32(2): 485–96.

Department of Health (1998a) *The New NHS – Modern, Dependable*. London: The Stationery Office.

Department of Health (1998b) *Commissioning in the New NHS, Health Service Circular 1998*. Department of Health: Leeds.

Fawcett, J. (1995) *Analysis and Evaluation of Conceptual Models of Nursing*, 3rd edn. Philadelphia: F.A. Davies.

Fawcett, J. (1999) The state of nursing science: hallmarks of the 20th and 21st centuries. *Nursing Science Quarterly* 12(4): 311–314.

Fawcett, J., Archer, C.L., Becker, D., Brown, K.K., Gann, S., Wong, M.J. and Wurster, A.B. (1992) Guidelines for selecting a conceptual model of nursing: focus on the individual patient. *Dimensions of Critical Care Nursing*. 11(5): 268–277.

Gibb, H. and Banfield, M. (1996) The issue of critical paths in Australia: where are they taking us? *Nursing Inquiry* 3(1): 36–44.

Gibson, T. and Heartfield, M. (1996) Critical pathways: A critical analysis. *International Journal of Nursing Practice* 2: 189–193.

Herring, L. (1999) Critical pathways: an efficient way to manage care. *Nursing Standard* 13(47): 11–17.

Holt, P., Wilson, A. and Ward, J. (1996) *Clinical Practice Guidelines and Critical Pathways: A Status Report on National and NSW Development and Implementation Activity*. Sydney: NSW Health Department.

Inatavicius, D.D. and Hausmann, K.A. (1995) *Clinical Pathways for Collaborative Practice*. Philadelphia: W.B. Saunders.

Ireson, C.L. (1997) Critical pathways: effectiveness in achieving patient outcomes. *Journal of Nursing Administration* 27(6):16–23.

Jaarsma, T. (1999) Developing a supportive-educative program for patients with advanced heart failure within Orem's General Theory of Nursing. In: Jaarsma, T. (ed) *Heart Failure: Nurses Care Effects of Education and Support by a Nurse on Self-Care, Resource Utilization and Quality of Life of Patients with Heart Failure*. Maastricht: Dadtwyse Maastricht.

Jaarsma, T., Halfens, R., Senten, M., Huijer, Abu-Sad, H. and Dracup, K. (1998) Developing a supportive-educative program for patients with advanced heart failure within Orem's General Theory of Nursing. *Nursing Science Quarterly* 11: 79–85.

Johnson, S. (1997a) Introduction to pathways of care. In: Johnson, S. (ed) *Pathways of Care* Oxford: Blackwell Science.

Johnson, S. (1997b) What is a pathway of care? In: Johnson, S. (ed) *Pathways of Care*. Oxford: Blackwell Science.

Johnson, S. (1997c) (ed) *Pathways of Care*. Oxford, Blackwell Science.

Jones, J. and Tucker, S. (2000) Exploring continuity and change. In: Brechin, A., Brown, H. and Eby, M. (eds) *Critical Practice in Health and Social Care*. London: Sage Publications.

Kitchiner, D., Davidson, C. and Bundred, P. (1996) Integrated care pathways: effective tools of continuous evaluation of clinical practice. *Journal of Evaluation in Clinical Practice* 2: 65–69.

Kwan, J. and Sandercock, P. (1999) In-hospital care pathways for stroke. In: *Cochrane Library* Issue 1, 2003, Oxford: Update Software, 36–37.

Mason, C. (1999) Guide to practice or 'load of rubbish'? The influence of care plans on nursing practice in five clinical areas in Northern Ireland. *Journal of Advanced Nursing* 29(2): 380–387.

McSherry, R., Simmons, M. and Pearce, P. (2002) An introduction to evidence-informed nursing. In: McSherry, R., Simmons, M. and Abbott, P. (eds) *Evidence-Informed Nursing: A Guide for Clinical Nurses*. London: Routledge Press.

Lee, T.T., Yeh, C. and Ho, L. (2002) Application of a computerized nursing care plan system in one hospital: experiences of ICU nurses in Taiwan. *Journal of Advanced Nursing* 39(1): 61, 67.

National Health Service (2003a) *National electronic Library for Protocols and Care Pathways*. (Online). Available at www.nehl.nhs.uk/carepathways/ (accessed 2 May, 2003).

National Health Service (2003b) *National electronic Library for Health*. (Online). Available at www.nehl.nhs.uk/ (accessed 2 May, 2003).

National Pathways Association (2003) *National Pathways Association*. Available at www.the.npa.org.uk/ (accessed 1 April, 2003).

Orem, D.E. (1971, 1980, 1985, 1995, 2001) *Nursing: Concepts of Practice*, 1st, 2nd, 3rd, 4th 5th and 6th edns. London: Mosby.

Pearson, A., Vaughan, B. and Fitzgerald, M. (2001) *Nursing Models for Practice*, 2nd edn. London: Butterworth Heinemann.

Polanczyk, C.A. and Lee, T.H. (2001) Potential pitfalls in the development of successful critical pathways. In: Cannon, C.P. and O'Gara, P.T. (eds) *Critical Pathways in Cardiology*. Philadelphia: Lippincott Williams and Wilkins.

Renholm, M., Leino-Kilpi, H. and Suominen, T. (2002) Critical pathways: A systematic review. *Journal of Nursing Administration* 32(4): 196–202.

Riley K. (1998) Paving the way. *Health Service Journal* 108: 30–31.

Scott, M. (2002) Critical pathways: aiming for seamless care. In: Hatchett, R. and Thompson, D. (eds) *Cardiac Nursing: A Comprehensive Guide*. London: Churchill Livingstone.

Stead, L. and Huckle, S. (1997) Pathways in cardiology. In: Johnson, S. (ed) *Pathways of Care*. Oxford: Blackwell Science.

Taylor, S.G. (2002) Dorothea E. Orem Self-care deficit theory of nursing. In: Alligood, M.R. and Marriner-Tomey, A. (eds) *Nursing Theory Utilisation & Application*. London: Mosby.

Walsh, M. (1998) *Models and Critical Pathways in Clinical Nursing*, 2nd edn. London: Baillière Tindall.

Wall, D. and Proyect, M.M. (1998) *Moving from Parameters to Pathways: A Guide for Developing and Implementing Critical Pathways*. Chicago: Precept Press.

Wammack, L., and Mabrey, J. D. (1999) Outcomes Assessment of Total Hip and Total Knee Arthroplasty: Critical Pathways, Variance Analysis, and Continuous Quality Improvement. *Clinical Nurse Specialist* 12(3): 122–129.

Williams, S. and Ramos, M.C. (1993) Mitral valve prolapse and its effects: a programme of inquiry within Orem's Self-Care Deficit Theory of nursing. *Journal of Advanced Nursing* 18: 742–751.

Chapter 3

Care plans for specific cardiac conditions

Key points

- Orem's (2001) conceptual model of nursing may be used to assess, plan and implement nursing care in the CCU.
- Case studies are presented to provide examples of application of Orem's (2001) conceptual model to individuals with cardiac conditions.
- The case studies and care plan examples provide guidelines for developing local care plans and use and are not definitive prescriptions for care.

Introduction

Nurses considering improving or developing conceptual models in their practice setting may require a visual guide to assist them with formulating assessment and planning documentation. As mentioned in the previous chapter, there is a dearth of information on the practical application of conceptual models of nursing in coronary care.

This chapter aims to provide some guidance on the use of Orem's (2001) conceptual model in the context of particular case histories (which do not relate to particular individuals). It is recommended that the reader refer to the original texts (Orem 1971, 1980, 1985, 1995, 2001) and other texts that describe the model (Fawcett 1995, Meleis 1997, Alligood and Marriner-Tomey 2002) for more detailed information.

One difficulty with case description and care planning for specific conditions is the variety of treatment interventions available for cardiac conditions both nationally and internationally. The proceeding care plans, therefore, are examples of how assessment and documentation *may* be used in nursing practice. They are not definitive plans for treating individual cases.

Patients with acute myocardial infarction (AMI), unstable angina and chronic heart failure are usually (although not exclusively) cared for in a coronary care unit (CCU). In some areas, patients who are deemed stable or uncomplicated are nursed in general wards as opposed to a small specialised coronary care unit. Nursing care in the CCU for individuals with these conditions should be planned in accordance with local, national and international standards, in relation to the best and current practice when caring for this patient group.

While other health professionals address the needs of the patients in specific areas such as provision of medical care, dietary and ambulatory needs, the nurse's plan represents an integration of the multiplicity of interventions that a patient may receive including the wider health issues such as psychosocial needs and places these within the framework of care. The plan is based on astute assessment of the patient's health needs and it is constructed in conjunction with patient and family or significant others (referred to generically as family) as appropriate.

Planning nursing care for individuals who have sustained a myocardial infarction

Conceptual-model-based care planning requires a good knowledge of the inherent framework of the model and underlying philosophy and theory. Planning for care using Orem's (2001) model of self-care requires that an initial assessment be carried out to ascertain the individual's demands for self-care, the inability to meet these self-care demands, the reason for self-care deficit and the potential for re-establishing self-care. This technique is used to assess the individual's usual routine and the problems that exist at present and impede self-care (Pearson et al. 2001). The patient's abilities are assessed to ascertain whether there are deficits to carry out self-care in each of the three areas where self-care requisites occur (universal requisites, health deviation requisites and developmental requisites) (Figure 3.1). The assessment identifies problems and needs that form the basis of the subsequent care plan. Measurement, observation and information from both the patient and their family inform each of the assessment categories.

This chapter presents three fictitious case histories pertaining to common cardiac conditions (myocardial infarction, acute heart failure and angioplasty). The care plans may be used as templates to develop similar documents tailored to nurses' local conditions and requirements.

Case history 1: A gentleman presenting with acute myocardial infarction

Mr Robert Smith is a 56-year-old gentleman who is transferred to the CCU from the emergency department approximately 30 minutes after arriving at the hospital. On admission, his wife, Julie, accompanies Mr Smith. He is very anxious and still has some pain. He has an intravenous (IV) line in place. IV morphine was given in the emergency department to relieve pain. Aspirin (300 mg) was also given. External blood pressure is recorded as 100/60 mmHg, pulse rate is 90 beats per minute (bpm). He is short of breath, his respiratory rate is 26 per minute and oxygen is being given continuously through a mask. He is perspiring, pale in colour and appears anxious.

An electrocardiograph (ECG) performed in the emergency department reveals a heart rate of 90 bpm with a normal sinus rhythm. The ECG reveals changes consistent with myocardial infarction. Because of the relevant history and typical ECG changes, Mr Smith received reperfusion therapy (thrombolysis) in the emergency department and subsequently a heparin infusion was started.

Background: Mr Smith is a self-employed carpenter with no previous history

Please indicate the extent to which the current admission has impacted upon the following self-care requisites:

Universal self-care requisites   Impact of condition:
  1. Maintaining a sufficient intake of air
  2. Maintaining a sufficient intake of water
  3. Maintaining a sufficient intake of food
  4. Providing care associated with elimination processes and excrements
  5. Maintaining a balance between solitude and rest
  6. Maintaining a balance between solitude and social interaction
  7. Preventing hazards to human life, human functioning, and wellbeing
  8. Promoting human functioning and development within social groups in accord with human potential, known human limitations and the human desire to be normal

Health deviation self-care requisites
  1. Seeking and securing appropriate medical assistance
  2. Being aware of and attending to the effects and results of pathological conditions and states
  3. Effectively carrying out medically prescribed measures
  4. Being aware of and attending to or regulating the discomforting or deleterious effects of medical care measures
  5. Modifying the self-concept in accepting oneself as being in a particular state of health and in need of special forms of healthcare
  6. Learning to live with the effects of health state and treatment in a lifestyle that promotes continued personal development

Developmental self-care requisites
  1. Seek to understand and form habits of introspection and reflection to develop insights about oneself and others
  2. Seek to accept feelings and emotions as leading, after reflection on them, to insights about self and about relationships with others
  3. Use talents and interests in preparing for and in maintaining and supporting engagement in productive work in society
  4. Engage in clarification of goals and values in situations that demand personal involvement
  5. Act with responsibility in life situations in accordance with one's role or roles
  6. Seek to understand the value of positive emotions
  7. Seek to understand that negative emotions and action impulses are experienced when conduct is in discord with one's life goals and self-ideal
  8. Promote positive mental health through deliberate efforts to function within a veridical (reality) frame of reference
  9. Function to bring about and maintain order in daily living
  10. Function with integrity
  11. Function as a person in community
  12. Function with increasing understanding of one's own humanity

Figure 3.1 Example of self-care deficits assessment documentation.

Adapted from Orem, D.E. (2001) *Nursing: Concepts of Practice* (6th edn). London: Mosby.

of cardiac disease and no previous admissions to hospital. He smokes 40 cigarettes per day.

In order to adequately plan for Mr Smith's care it is important to have an understanding of the underlying condition, myocardial infarction. A brief outline of the condition and treatment is provided here. Key texts on the subject such as Jowett and Thompson (2000) and Hatchett and Thompson (2002) are recommended for further details.

Myocardial infarction

Coronary heart disease is a major cause of premature death in the world (Quinn et al. 2002). Individuals with this condition usually develop atherosclerotic plaques in the coronary arteries. These narrow the diameter of the coronary arteries, thereby reducing essential blood flow to the heart muscle. In some cases the individual may be symptom free. In other cases there may be chest pain (angina pectoris) due to partial obstruction (ischaemia) of the coronary arteries or there may be complete coronary artery obstruction resulting in destruction and cell death (necrosis) in the cardiac muscle (myocardium) – myocardial infarction (MI).

MI is an acute condition that requires hospitalisation and accounts for a large number of out-of-hospital deaths (Norris 1998). It also accounts for the majority of deaths from coronary heart disease (Quinn et al. 2002). This event occurs due to prolonged reduction of blood flow to the heart muscle (myocardium) due to thrombus formation and platelet aggregation occluding blood flow through a coronary artery, which is usually associated with pre-existing atherosclerotic plaques (Quinn et al. 2002). These plaques can contribute to the thrombus formation as they can rupture or crack (fissure), which activates the body's clotting mechanisms.

Patients usually present with what Quinn et al. (2002) describe as the 'classic symptoms' of MI, although the symptoms can vary and there is increasing evidence that women's presentation may be different from that of men. The classic symptoms include: severe central 'crushing' chest pain, lasting for more than 30 minutes, and is not relieved (at home or in hospital) by administration of sublingual nitrate preparations (glyceryl trinitrate (GTN)) This pain often extends to the jaw, neck, back or shoulders and may be accompanied by nausea and/or vomiting. The autonomic nervous system may be affected, resulting in profuse sweating, with the patient appearing cold and clammy (Quinn et al. 2002).

If the reduced blood flow persists for more than 2 hours there may be permanent damage to the myocardium with related loss of function. The focus of hospital care in the immediate phase is on accurate and speedy diagnosis, pain relief, reperfusion of the obstructed areas of the heart, limiting the size of the infarction, prevention/detection/treatment of complications, and providing the patient and their family with information and support.

Once the patient is admitted to the hospital diagnosis of MI is established by the physician or nurse-led service (in collaboration with a physician). The patient's presenting condition is an important indicator and a full physical examination is essential. The staff question the patient/family regarding the history of onset, duration and type of pain to create an accurate picture of the presenting condition. In addition, presence of sweating, nausea and vomiting are noted. A 12-lead ECG is crucial for diagnosis as is the presence of biochemical cardiac 'markers' in the blood (such as creatine kinase, troponins T and I), which provide a clear physiological indication that an infarction has taken place.

The initial assessment, which may take place in the community setting, emergency department or hospital ward, depending on the circumstances, must be performed with minimum time wastage to ensure that the patient's condition is diagnosed quickly and they receive prompt treatment. The history and physical examination are considered in conjunction with the results of ECG and laboratory blood tests to confirm a diagnosis of MI.

Once the diagnosis of myocardial infarction is established, prompt treatment aims to re-establish blood supply to the myocardium thereby reducing the effects of the infarction. Thrombolytic agents such as streptokinase, tPA (tisssue plasminogen activator) and reteplase are commonly administrated to dissolve the thrombus, if there are no contraindications (Connaughton 2001). Immediate re-establishment of the blood supply is often undertaken by invasive techniques (angioplasty), which is a standard treatment for atherosclerosis and is becoming increasingly common in the treatment of acute coronary syndromes in some cardiac units. The faster reperfusion commences the better the outcome. The UK standards recommend that suitable individuals should receive therapy within 60 minutes of calling for professional help, and similar guidelines exist in other countries throughout the world (Department of Health 2000).

Thrombolysis therapy was traditionally administered in the CCU. However, quick administration is essential to limit the effect of the MI and therapy is increasingly being given in the emergency department and in the community (Quinn 1999). Aspirin therapy (reduces platelet function thereby preventing thrombus formation) is usually given in conjunction with this as it reduces mortality, even when used without thrombolysis (ISIS-2 1988). Newer anti-platelet drugs are also commonly used.

Admission to the CCU facilitates intensive monitoring of the patient's condition, as there are usually small numbers of patients, a high staff–patient ratio and specialised technological equipment to support close monitoring. This also facilitates close physical observation of the patient and prompt intervention in emergency situations.

Due to the effect of the MI on cardiac structure and function, major life-threatening complications can occur that require immediate treatment and the healthcare staff monitor the patient closely for these events. These include abnormalities of cardiac rhythm and failure of the heart pumping mechanism (ventricular failure).

Pain control is another priority for MI patients while in the CCU. Opiate analgesia such as diamorphine or morphine is used to relieve the severe pain associated with the event in addition to IV nitrates that reduce ischaemic pain through reduction of cardiac workload. In addition, breathing is closely monitored and oxygen therapy is given in the initial stages to improve oxygen supply to the myocardium, which may be reduced due to impaired heart function. This is to maintain adequate oxygen saturation of above 95% and may be reduced as the condition improves.

Planning the care

Planning Mr Smith's care using Orem's (2001) model of self-care requires that an initial assessment to ascertain this gentleman's demands for self-care, his inability to meet these demands, the reason for self-care deficit and the potential for re-establishing self-care.

From this assessment (Figure 3.2), self-care deficits were identified in the areas of

Please indicate the extent to which the current admission has impacted upon the following self-care requisites:

Universal self-care requisites

1. Maintaining a sufficient intake of air

Impact of condition: myocardial infarction
Rate of breathing: 26
Oxygen saturation level: 90%
Not tolerating fluids at present
Nausea at present

2. Maintaining a sufficient intake of water
3. Maintaining a sufficient intake of food
4. Providing care associated with elimination processes and excrements

Potential of constipation due to bed rest, unable to toilet unassisted

5. Maintaining a balance between solitude and rest

Needs to have rest following cardiac event
Needs support of friends and family

6. Maintaining a balance between solitude and social interaction
7. Preventing hazards to human life, human functioning and well-being

Fatigued, usually likes to play golf
Potential of life-threatening cardiac arrhythmias
Chest pain present on admission
BP 110/60; pulse: 90; is a smoker

8. Promoting human functioning and development within social groups in accord with human potential, known human limitations and the human desire to he normal

Lives with his wife in house in suburban area. Enjoys his work, although believes this to be under threat due to his hospital admission

Health deviation self-care requisites

1. Seeking and securing appropriate medical assistance

Woke up with pain during the night, with chest pain, which became so severe that he had to call an ambulance. Usually refers to GP

2. Being aware of and attending to the effects and results of pathological conditions and states

Aware of some effects of condition, but unable to attend to these

3. Effectively carrying out medically prescribed measures
4. Being aware of and attending to or regulating the discomforting or deleterious effects of medical care measures

Receiving thrombolysis, oxygen and analgesia
Unaware of potential deleterious effects of medical care measures and unable to attend or regulate in the event of it

5. Modifying the self-concept in accepting oneself as being in a particular state of health and in need of special forms of healthcare

Unaware of potential outcome of diagnosis and treatment

6. Learning to live with the effects of health state and treatment in a lifestyle that promotes continued personal development

Unaware of potential health effects of myocardial infarction or lifestyle changes that may be necessary

Developmental self-care requisites

1. Seek to understand and form habits of introspection and reflection to develop insights about oneself and others
   — This major event has prompted introspection and reflection. In particular provoking reflection upon lifestyles such as smoking and its impact on health

2. Seek to accept feelings and emotions as leading, after reflection on them, to insights about self and about relationships with others
   — Emotions present: anger, sadness, however, little reflection on these yet

3. Use talents and interests in preparing for and in maintaining and supporting engagement in productive work in society
   — Work temporarily halted due to condition

4. Engage in clarification of goals and values in situations that demand personal involvement
   — Withdrawn from usual life situations at present

5. Act with responsibility in life situations in accordance with one's role or roles
   — Role diminished temporarily due to hospitalisation

6. Seek to understand the value of positive emotions
   — Positive emotion of relief and happiness to be alive present, little understanding of the value of these given the current context, overwhelmed by negative emotions

7. Seek to understand that negative emotions and action impulses are experienced when conduct is in discord with one's life goals and self-ideal.
   — Negative emotions present, too shocked to begin to understand them

8. Promote positive mental health through deliberate efforts to function within a veridical (reality) frame of reference
   — Very anxious about current condition

9. Function to bring about and maintain order in daily living
   — Order in living dictated by hospital routine at present

10. Function with integrity
    — Able to function with integrity

11. Function as a person in community
    — Not living in usual community at present – hospitalised

12. Function with increasing understanding of one's own humanity
    — This experience has precipitated a belief of his personal 'frailty' as a human

Figure 3.2 Assessment of Mr Smith's self-care deficits.

Adapted from Orem, D.E. (2001) *Nursing: Concepts of Practice* (6th edn). London: Mosby.

preventing hazards to human life, human functioning and wellbeing; maintaining a sufficient intake of air; knowledge deficit with regard to maintenance of oxygenation; maintaining a sufficient intake of water; maintaining a sufficient intake of food; providing care associated with elimination processes and excrements; maintaining a balance between solitude and social interaction and human functioning and development within social groups; being aware of and attending to the effects and results of pathological conditions and states; effectively carrying out medically prescribed measures and learning to live with the effects of health state and treatment in a lifestyle that promotes continued personal development. These self-care deficits form the basis of the subsequent care plan (Table 3.1)

The nursing actions set out in the care plan aim to address Mr Smith's self-care deficits and enable him to meet his universal, health deviation and developmental requisites. In the early stages of his condition the nursing actions are wholly compensatory: acting for and doing for Mr Smith, things that he is unable to do for himself due to his condition. This involves providing physical and psychological support, guiding and directing and providing and maintaining an environment that supports personal development.

As Mr Smith's condition improves the nursing actions will be reviewed on the care plan, and may become partially compensatory as he is supported and encouraged to do for himself as his condition allows. This increases his independence, improves his confidence and prepares him for his return to self-care after discharge. Increasingly, nursing actions will focus on providing guidance, direction and teaching as Mr Smith is prepared for discharge and associated self-care deficits are addressed (see Table 3.1). Teaching is a crucial aspect of care for Mr Smith, as self-care deficits exist with regard to knowledge of his condition, his need to use medication and the need to live in a way that fosters his continued development. Teaching in the CCU focuses on describing the condition, taking prescribed medication (and possible side-effects), returning to usual activity level, preventing and treating further symptoms and managing risk factors for coronary heart disease. Family involvement in this teaching is essential. Risk factor management and cardiac patient education are discussed in more detail in Chapters 4 and 5.

Planning nursing care for individuals who have unstable angina

Unstable angina is a medical emergency that requires management in the CCU (Quinn et al. 2002).

Case history 2: A lady presenting with unstable angina

Mrs Catherine Blake is a 60-year-old lady who is transferred to the CCU from the emergency department and is accompanied by her husband, following a 24-hour history of worsening chest pain. An IV line is in place. Mrs Blake had severe chest pain on admission to the emergency department and IV morphine was administered. IV nitrate therapy was commenced and aspirin 300 mg (oral) was also given. Her blood pressure is recorded as 150/80 mmHg, and her pulse rate is 105 bpm. Her respiratory rate is 22 per minute and oxygen is being given

Table 3.1 Care plan for Mr Smith

Self-care deficit	Goal	Specific nursing actions	Description of general nursing actions	Review instructions (reduce as condition improves)
Preventing hazards to human life, human functioning, and wellbeing	Treatment of hazard to human life (myocardial infarction)	Observe patient for adverse effects of this thrombolytic and anticoagulant therapy (including bleeding, haemorrhage and sensitivity) Assess pain level and provide analgesia (diamorphine/morphine) Intravenous nitrate therapy if required/prescribed Inotrope therapy if required Advise regarding cautions with oxgyen	Providing physical support	Observe for adverse effects hourly Evaluate pain hourly
	Observe effectiveness of treatment	Record ECG following thrombolysis to assess effectiveness of therapy Evaluate effectiveness of analgesia	Providing physical support	Review ECG following thrombolysis Evaluate effectiveness of analgesia hourly
	Early detection of hazards to human life	Continuous ECG monitoring to detect life-threatening arrhythmias Management of arrhythmias Monitoring and reporting of ST-segment changes to observe for extension of infarction Management of subsequent infarction Monitoring and reporting of early signs of heart failure Management of heart failure Assess blood pressure and pulse rate Maintenance of patency and hygiene of intravenous line Monitoring and reporting electrolyte levels and administering treatment as prescribed	Providing physical support	Continuous evaluation through monitoring Hourly review of blood pressure

Table 3.1 *continued*

Self-care deficit	Goal	Specific nursing actions	Description of general nursing actions	Review instructions (reduce as condition improves)
Maintaining a sufficient intake of air	To ensure optimum oxygen intake	Administer oxygen Monitoring oxygen saturations continuously Monitor respiratory rate hourly Observe colour for signs of cyanosis Observe breathing pattern for regularity and signs of breathlessness	Providing physical support	Review respiratory status hourly As condition improves oxygen may be reduced and/or removed
	To reduce myocardial oxygen demand	Maintain on bed rest for at least 4 hours, with gradual return to normal activity level over 2–6 weeks depending on condition Restrict activity in initial 24 hours	Guiding and directing	Review daily Activity level may be increased slowly as condition improves
Knowledge deficit with regard to maintenance of oxygenation	To ensure that rationale for care is understood	Explanation of processes of myocardial infarction and subsequent need for oxygen Explanation of rationale for rest and reduced activity Provide heart booklets and reading material to support information given	Teaching Guiding and directing	Review daily Teaching may be reinforced if deficits persist
Maintaining a sufficient intake of water	To prevent fluid overload	Provide moderate fluids once nausea and vomiting ceases Monitor and record accurate fluid intake and output Implement measures to maintain adequate fluid balance	Providing physical support	Review hourly
Maintaining a sufficient intake of food	To provide adequate nutrition	Administer anti-emetics to reduce nausea and vomiting Provide light appetising meals once nausea and vomiting cease	Acting for or doing for another	Review daily

Providing care associated with elimination processes and excrements	To provide assistance with elimination while activity is restricted	Provide assistance when using elimination facilities while activity is restricted. Provide assistance with hygiene needs while activity is restricted. Ensure patient's dignity is maintained and appropriate level of self-care	Acting for or doing for another	Review daily
Maintaining a balance between solitude and social interaction	To facilitate balance between solitude and social interaction while hospitalised	Facilitate visiting of family and provide family facilities as appropriate. Ensure that patient receives adequate periods of rest	Providing psychological support. Providing and maintaining an environment that supports personal development	Review daily
Human functioning and development within social groups	To acknowledge the temporary loss of normal social role and to provide support	Demonstrate empathy and understanding of Mr Smith's feelings in this situation. Ensure maintenance of family contacts. Foster Mr Smith's sense of self	Providing psychological support. Providing and maintaining an environment that supports personal development	Review daily
Being aware of and attending to the effects and results of pathological conditions and states	To ensure that the condition of myocardial infarction is understood upon discharge	Explanation of the anatomy and physiology of the heart. Explanation of pathology of myocardial infarction. Explanation of causes and results of myocardial infarction. Provide booklets and reading material to support information given. Obtaining a blood lipid profile and ensuring treatment and advice for raised levels if appropriate	Teaching. Guiding and directing	Evaluate explanations daily. Review at discharge
Effectively carrying out medically prescribed measures	To ensure that Mr Smith understands medication requirements upon discharge	Explanation of the reason for medication being prescribed. Explanation of the medication action and effects. Explanation of time of timing, dosage and mode of administration of medication. Relevant teaching of medication administration if required. Explanation of the importance of taking medication on time. Explain potential side-effects of medication. Provide information on whom to contact if side-effects to medication occur	Teaching. Guiding and directing	Evaluate explanations daily. Review at discharge

Table 3.1 *continued*

Self-care deficit	Goal	Specific nursing actions	Description of general nursing actions	Review instructions (reduce as condition improves)
Learning to live with the effects of health state and treatment in a lifestyle that promotes continued personal development	To support Mr Smith's rehabilitation	Explain the necessity for gradual re-establishment of previous activity level Ensure that Mr Smith is registered in a cardiac rehabilitation programme or equivalent Teaching and explanation about the importance of lifestyle modification (including smoking cessation) to improve health		Evaluate explanations daily Review at discharge

Adapted from Orem, D.E. (2001) *Nursing: Concepts of Practice* (6th edn). London: Mosby.

continuously through a mask. She is pale in colour and is still experiencing chest pain.

An ECG performed in the emergency department reveals ischaemic changes consistent with unstable angina.

Background: Mrs Blake is a factory worker with no previous history of cardiac disease and no previous admissions to hospital. She smokes 20 cigarettes per day.

Unstable angina

In the presence of atherosclerosis, angina is the term used to describe the discomfort that occurs during disruption in blood supply through coronary artery/ies. It can also occur in the absence of atherosclerosis due to coronary artery spasm. In either case insufficient oxygen to meet the requirements of the heart muscle (myocardium) results in an imbalance between supply and demand and there is pain due to this ischaemia, known as angina (Quinn et al. 2002).

Very often angina presents when there is an additional demand on the workload of the heart. Any factor that causes an increase in the heart rate increases the workload. This may be exercise, exertion, walking up a hill, carrying a bag, stress or physiological factors. The relationship between the increased demand and the ischaemic pain depends on many factors, including the severity of the underlying disease. Stable angina involves atherosclerosis of one or more coronary arteries that is fairly consistent and stable, causing a reduction in blood supply during times of extra demand (Quinn et al. 2002).

Unstable angina occurs due to rupture of an atherosclerotic plaque, formation of micro-thrombi at the rupture site and intermittent obstruction of the coronary artery. The classic symptoms include recent onset of angina symptoms (between 4 and 6 weeks), a change in usual symptoms (increased severity or occasions or less responsive to nitrates) and pain or discomfort during minimal exertion or rest (Quinn et al. 2002). This situation requires immediate medical attention to prevent progression to total occlusion of the artery (MI) or arrhythmias due to ischaemia, which can occur in up to 30% of cases (Quinn et al. 2002).

Diagnosis of unstable angina is established initially by history, physical examination and a 12-lead ECG (Connaughton 2001). Although the symptoms may be similar to AMI, there is no evidence of irreversible myocardial damage. Treatment aims to stabilise condition, relieve the symptoms and prevent further thrombus formation and possible MI. Medical treatment consists of anti-ischaemic therapy, anti-coagulant therapy, anti-platelet therapy and symptom relief (Connaughton 2001). Beta-blockers and nitrates are the mainstay of treatment. Nitrates are given IV initially and titrated to relieve pain. Anti-coagulant therapy (IV heparin) is required for 2–5 days. Low molecular weight heparins such as enoxaparin are being used increasingly. All patients receive aspirin therapy (75 mg once daily) unless contraindicated. Antiplatelet therapy may be given in place of anti-coagulant therapy, especially where contraindications are present.

Symptom relief is achieved by oxygen therapy to maintain oxygen saturation of above 95%. Opiate analgesics such as diamorphine or morphine are used to relieve the severe pain associated with the event. Rest in the CCU is also important. Once the condition has stabilised risk profiling and further investigations may be carried out to determine the extent of disease. This may include echocardiography, exercise stress testing and coronary angiographies. Further management of the patient depends on the results of these investigations. Usually local centres discuss individual cases to determine the level of risk associated with their condition. Future management may include pharmacological treatment, lifestyle modification and possible angioplasty and stent insertion or coronary artery bypass grafting depending on the extent of disease and the individual patient's case.

Planning the care

Planning Mrs Blake's care using Orem's (2001) model of self-care requires that an initial assessment be carried out to ascertain this lady's demands for self-care, her inability to meet these self-care demands, the reason for self-care deficit and the potential for re-establishing self-care.

Mrs Blake's assessment (Figure 3.3), reveals self-care deficits in the areas of preventing hazards to human life, human functioning and human wellbeing; maintaining a sufficient intake of air; providing care associated with elimination processes and excrements; maintaining a balance between solitude and social interaction and human functioning and development within social groups; being aware of and attending to the effects and results of pathological conditions and states; effectively carrying out medically prescribed measures; learning to live with the effects of health state and treatment in a lifestyle that promotes continued personal development and seeking to understand and form habits of introspection and reflection to develop insights about oneself and others. These self-care deficits form the basis of the subsequent care plan (Table 3.2).

The nursing actions set out in the care plan aim to address Mrs Blake's self-care deficits and enable her to meet her universal, health deviation and developmental requisites. In the early stages of her condition the nursing actions are wholly compensatory: acting for and doing for Mrs Blake, things that she is unable to do for herself due to her condition. This involves providing physical and psychological support, guiding and directing and providing and maintaining an environment that supports personal development.

As Mrs Blake's condition improves nursing actions will be reviewed on the care plan, and may become partially compensatory as she is supported and encouraged to do for herself as her condition allows. Increasingly nursing actions will focus on providing guidance, direction and teaching as Mrs Blake is prepared for discharge and/or subsequent invasive treatment (angioplasty or coronary artery bypass surgery) and associated self-care deficits are addressed (see Figure 3.3). As Mrs Blake is an identified high-risk candidate for the development of a major cardiovascular event, teaching and support will focus primarily upon risk factor management. It is essential that she understand her condition, subsequent treatment and prescribed medication. To enable her to live life to its full potential, it is essential that a systematic and rigorous approach to risk factor management is achieved. This may include assessment of her risk factors, readiness to learn and information needs. She may also be referrred to specialist services for smoking cessation. Family involvement is also essential. See Chapters 4 and 5 for risk factor managment and patient education.

Please indicate the extent to which the current admission has impacted upon the following self-care requisites:

Universal self-care requisites	
1. Maintaining a sufficient intake of air	Impact of condition: unstable angina
	Rate of breathing: 22
	Oxygen saturation level: 95%
2. Maintaining a sufficient intake of water	Drinking well
3. Maintaining a sufficient intake of food	Appetite poor at present
4. Providing care associated with elimination processes and excrements	Potential of constipation due to bed rest, unable to toilet unassisted
5. Maintaining a balance between solitude and rest	Needs to have rest following cardiac event
	Needs support of friends and family
6. Maintaining a balance between solitude and social interaction	Fatigued, likes playing cards and socialising
7. Preventing hazards to human life, human functioning and wellbeing	Potential of life-threatening cardiac arrhythmias
	Presence of chest pain
	Potential of myocardial infarction, is a smoker
8. Promoting human functioning and development within social groups in accord with human potential, known human limitations and the human desire to be normal	Enjoys working and socialising with work friends. Reduced function in social groups due to hospitalisation. Lives with her husband in an apartment in the city
Health deviation self-care requisites	
1. Seeking and securing appropriate medical assistance	Sought emergency care due to persistent severe chest pain, usually visits GP
2. Being aware of and attending to the effects and results of pathological conditions and states	Aware of some effects of condition, but unable to attend to these
3. Effectively carrying out medically prescribed measures	Receiving oxygen and analgesia
4. Being aware of and attending to or regulating the discomforting or deleterious effects of medical care measures	Unaware of potential deleterious effects of medical care measures and unable to attend or regulate in the event of it
5. Modifying the self-concept in accepting oneself as being in a particular state of health and in need of special forms of healthcare	Unaware of potential outcome of diagnosis and treatment
6. Learning to live with the effects of health state and treatment in a lifestyle that promotes continued personal development	Unaware of potential health effects
Developmental self-care requisites	
1. Seek to understand and form habits of introspection and reflection to develop insights about oneself and others	Level of introspection and reflection undeveloped in relation to the condition and lifestyle and its impact on health
2. Seek to accept feelings and emotions as leading, after reflection on them, to insights about self and about relationships with others	Emotions present: fear, however, little reflection on feelings as yet
3. Use talents and interests in preparing for and in maintaining and supporting engagement in productive work in society	Work temporarily halted due to condition
4. Engage in clarification of goals and values in situations that demand personal involvement	Withdrawn from usual life situations at present
5. Act with responsibility in life situations in accordance with one's role or roles	Role diminished temporarily due to hospitalisation
6. Seek to understand the value of positive emotions	Positive emotion of relief to be receiving hospital care, little understanding the value of these given the current context, overwhelmed by negative emotions (fear)
7. Seek to understand that negative emotions and action impulses are experienced when conduct is in discord with one's life goals and self-ideal.	Understands origin of negative emotions (fear). This fear relates to social and personal function in society, which Mrs Blake believes may be reduced due to condition
8. Promote positive mental health through deliberate efforts to function within a veridical (reality) frame of reference	Very concerned about current condition
9. Function to bring about and maintain order in daily living	Order in living dictated by hospital routine at present
10. Function with integrity	Functioning with integrity within confines of hospital
11. Function as a person in community	Temporarily not functioning within community, and misses this
12. Function with increasing understanding of one's own humanity	This hospitalisation has prompted thoughts about Mrs Blake's humanity

Figure 3.3 Assessment of Mrs Blake's self-care deficits.

Adapted from Orem, D.E. (2001) *Nursing: Concepts of Practice* (6th edn). London: Mosby.

Table 3.2 Care plan for Mrs Blake

Self-care deficit	Goal	Specific nursing actions	Description of general nursing actions	Review instructions (reduce as condition improves)
Preventing hazards to human life, human functioning, and wellbeing	Treatment of hazard to human life (unstable angina)	Administer anticoagulant therapy (heparin) Observe patient for adverse effects of this therapy (including bleeding, haemorrhage and sensitivity) Assess pain level and provide analgesia (diamorphine/morphine) Intravenous nitrate therapy Beta-blocker therapy as prescribed Inotrope therapy if required Advise regarding cautions with oxgyen	Providing physical support	Observe for adverse effects hourly Evaluate pain hourly
	Early detection of hazards to human life	Continuous ECG monitoring to detect life-threatening arrhythmias Management of arrhythmias Monitoring and reporting of ST-segment changes to observe for possible myocardial infarction Management of subsequent infarction Assess blood pressure and pulse rate Maintenance of patency and hygiene of intravenous line	Providing physical support	Continuous evaluation through monitoring Hourly review of blood pressure
Maintaining a sufficient intake of air	To ensure optimum oxygen intake	Administer oxygen Monitoring oxygen saturations continuously Monitor respiratory rate hourly Observe colour for signs of cyanosis Observe breathing pattern for regularity and signs of breathlessness	Providing physical support	Review respiratory status hourly As condition improves oxygen may be reduced and/or removed
	To reduce myocardial oxygen demand	Maintain on bed rest for at least 4 hours, with gradual return to normal activity level over 2–6 weeks depending on condition Restrict activity in initial 24 hours	Guiding and directing	Review daily Activity level may be increased slowly as condition improves

Need	Objective	Nursing actions	Method	Evaluation
Providing care associated with elimination processes and excrements	To provide assistance with elimination while activity is restricted	Provide assistance when using elimination facilities while activity is restricted. Provide assistance with hygiene needs while activity is restricted. Ensure patient's dignity is maintained and appropriate level of self-care	Acting for or doing for another	Review daily
Maintaining a balance between solitude and social interaction	To facilitate balance between solitude and social interaction while hospitalised	Facilitate visiting of family and provide family facilities as appropriate. Ensure that patient receives adequate periods of rest	Providing psychological support. Providing and maintaining an environment that supports personal development	Review daily
Human functioning and development within social groups	To acknowledge the temporary loss of normal social role and to provide support	Demonstrate empathy and understanding of Mrs Blake's feelings in this situation. Ensure maintenance of family contacts. Foster Mrs Blake's sense of self	Providing psychological support. Providing and maintaining an environment that supports personal development	Review daily
Being aware of and attending to the effects and results of pathological conditions and states	To ensure that the condition of myocardial infarction is understood upon discharge	Explanation of the anatomy and physiology of the heart. Explanation of pathology of angina. Explanation of causes and results of angina. Provide booklets and reading material to support information given	Teaching. Guiding and directing	Evaluate explanations daily. Review at discharge
Effectively carrying out medically prescribed measures	To ensure that Mrs Blake understands medication requirements upon discharge	Explanation of the reason for medication being prescribed. Explanation of the medication action and effects. Explanation of timing, dosage and mode of administration of medication. Relevant teaching of medication administration if required. Explanation of the importance of taking medication on time. Explain potential side-effects of medication. Provide information on whom to contact if side effects to medication occur	Teaching. Guiding and directing	Evaluate explanations daily. Review at discharge

Table 3.2 continued

Self-care deficit	Goal	Specific nursing actions	Description of general nursing actions	Review instructions (reduce as condition improves)
Learning to live with the effects of health state and treatment in a lifestyle that promotes continued personal development	To encourage and facilitate adoption of a lifestyle that will promote health	Clear and specific teaching and explanation about the importance of lifestyle modification (including smoking cessation) to improve health Provide information and contacts for relevant support groups Provide information leaflets as appropriate Prepare for invasive treatments (angioplasty or bypass surgery) as appropriate		Evaluate explanations daily Review at discharge
Seek to understand and form habits of introspection and reflection to develop insights about oneself and others	To encourage and facilitate reflection on lifestyle and its implication for health	Explore Mrs Blake's understanding of lifestyle and its impact upon her own health Explore Mrs Blake's understanding and awareness of the contribution of smoking to the development of her own disease Explore Mrs Blake's willingness to change her behaviours in this area Referral to nurse-led clinic/cardiac rehabilitation		

Adapted from Orem, D.E. (2001) *Nursing: Concepts of Practice* (6th edn). London: Mosby.

Planning nursing care for individuals who have chronic heart failure

Chronic heart failure (CHF) is a common and debilitating condition (Gould 2002). While the mortality rate from coronary heart disease appears to be declining in Western countries, hospital admission for heart failure appear to be on the increase (Sharpe and Doughty 1998). This occurrence is described by McMurray and Stewart (2001) as 'the increasing burden of chronic heart failure'. The increase has been ascribed to the ever advancing treatment modalities for acute cardiac conditions such as MI, resulting in better survival rates, but the existence of a population that is susceptible to heart failure. McMurray and Stewart (2001: 1) describe this phenomenon as 'the residual effects of better health-care strategies'.

Case history 3: A lady with chronic heart failure

Mrs Jean Butler is a 72-year-old lady who was transferred to the CCU from the emergency department following an acute onset of shortness of breath and difficulty in breathing (dyspnoea) during the night approximately 30 minutes after arrival to the hospital. She is accompanied by her husband. She appears pale and her skin is cool and clammy. An IV line is in place. IV morphine was given in the emergency department to relieve pain. External blood pressure is recorded as 110/60 mmHg, pulse rate is 120 bpm. She is short of breath, her respiratory rate is 30 per minute and oxygen is being given continuously through a facemask. A diuretic, IV frusemide (furosemide) 40 mg was administered in the emergency department.

An ECG was also performed revealing sinus tachycardia (rate 120) and changes consistent with chronic heart failure.

Background: Mrs Butler is a retired schoolteacher who has had previous hospital admissions; once for an MI and one subsequent episode of acute heart failure. She is a non-smoker.

Chronic heart failure

The symptoms of CHF include exercise intolerance, dyspnoea, breathlessness, oedema and fatigue (Gould 2002). There are many reasons for the onset of the syndrome of CHF, and diseases such as coronary heart disease (CHD), cardiomyopathy, chronic hypertension, valvular dysfunction and infection are often contributory factors in development. CHD is the most common contributory factor (Gould 2002). The underlying physiological cause for heart failure is usually dysfunction of the left ventricle of the heart (Gould 2002).

CHF is a life-threatening condition associated with high mortality (McMurray and Stewart 2001). There is increasing impetus in the UK, Ireland, Australia and many parts of Europe to manage these patients through outpatient-based nurse-led clinics, not only to reduce the financial and other implications of hospitalisation, but also to improve outcome by providing a specialist monitoring and advice service round the clock and to improve quality of life by reduced hospitalisation and emotional support.

Diagnosis of CHF is confirmed by measures of ventricular structure and function including chest radiographs, 12-lead ECG, echocardiogram, radionuclide studies and laboratory blood tests. Although CHF is effectively treated in the community or hospital ward when the patient is acutely ill with compromised respiratory and cardiac status, CCU admission is indicated to stabilise the condition and initiate life-saving treatment if required. Treatment aims to improve symptoms and prevent death and includes intensive oxygen therapy, diuretic therapy, nitrate therapy, angiotensin-converting enzyme (ACE) inhibitors, rest, comfort measures and emotional support.

Opiate analgesics such as diamorphine or morphine are used to reduced cardiac workload. Oxygen therapy is given in the initial stages to improve oxygen supply to the myocardium, which may be reduced due to impaired heart function. This maintains adequate oxygen saturation of above 95%, which may be reduced as the condition improves. Admission to the CCU is required in most cases to facilitate the intensive monitoring that the condition requires. The high patient–staff ratio in most CCUs facilitates close observation of the patient and effect intervention in emergency situations.

Planning the care

Planning Mrs Butler's care using Orem's (2001) model of self-care requires an initial assessment to ascertain this lady's demands for self-care, her inability to meet these self-care demands, the reason for self-care deficit and the potential for re-establishing self-care.

Mrs Blake's assessment (Figure 3.4), reveals self-care deficits in the areas of preventing hazards to human life, human functioning and human wellbeing; maintaining a sufficient intake of air and water; providing care associated with elimination processes and excrements; maintaining a balance between solitude and social interaction and human functioning and development within social groups; being aware of and attending to the effects and results of pathological conditions and states; effectively carrying out medically prescribed measures and learning to live with the effects of health state and treatment in a lifestyle that promotes continued personal development. These self-care deficits form the basis of the subsequent care plan (Table 3.3).

The nursing actions set out in the care plan aim to address Mrs Butler's self-care deficits and enable her to meet her universal, health deviation and developmental requisites. In the early stages of her condition the nursing actions are wholly compensatory: acting for and doing for Mrs Butler, things that she is unable to do for herself due to her condition. This involves providing physical and psychological support, guiding and directing and providing and maintaining an environment that supports personal development.

As Mrs Butler's condition improves nursing actions will be reviewed on the care plan, and may become partially compensatory as she is supported and encouraged to do for herself as her condition allows. Increasingly nursing actions will focus on providing guidance, direction and teaching as Mrs Butler is prepared for discharge and associated self-care deficits are addressed (see Table 3.3). Preparing Mrs Butler for self-care upon discharge is a crucial aspect of the nursing action. Heart failure is

Please indicate the extent to which the current admission has impacted upon the following self-care requisites:

Universal self-care requisites	Impact of condition: myocardial infarction
1. Maintaining a sufficient intake of air	Rate of breathing: 30 Oxygen saturation level: 90%
2. Maintaining a sufficient intake of water	Not tolerating fluids at present. Weight 52.6 kg (116 lbs)
3. Maintaining a sufficient intake of food	Nausea present
4. Providing care associated with elimination processes and excrements	Potential of constipation due to bed rest, unable to toilet unassisted
5. Maintaining a balance between solitude and rest	Needs to have rest following cardiac event Needs support of friends and family
6. Maintaining a balance between solitude and social interaction	Enjoys solitary hobbies such as painting and reading
7. Preventing hazards to human life, human functioning, and wellbeing	Potential of life threatening heart failure
8. Promoting human functioning and development within social groups in accord with human potential, known human limitations and the human desire to he normal	Lives with her husband in a large suburban house Maintains contact with some work colleagues

Health deviation self-care requisites	
1. Seeking and securing appropriate medical assistance	Woke up with breathlessness during the night, which became so severe that she had to call an ambulance
2. Being aware of and attending to the effects and results of pathological conditions and states	Receiving oxygen and analgesia
3. Effectively carrying out medically prescribed measures	Unaware of potential deleterious effects of medical care measures and unable to attend or regulate in the event of it
4. Being aware of and attending to or regulating the discomforting or deleterious effects of medical care measures	Unaware of potential outcome of diagnosis and treatment
5. Modifying the self-concept in accepting oneself as being in a particular state of health and in need of special forms of healthcare	Understands that she has suffered from 'heart problems' and requires medication
6. Learning to live with the effects of health state and treatment in a lifestyle that promotes continued personal development	Understands that medication is important to maintaining her health

Developmental self-care requisites	
1. Seek to understand and form habits of introspection and reflection to develop insights about oneself and others	Currently, reflecting upon this disorder and its impact potential impact upon her life in order to develop insights about how she may change her lifestyle to adapt
2. Seek to accept feelings and emotions as leading, after reflection on them, to insights about self and about relationships with others	Accepts emotions and feelings as an essential part of life
3. Use talents and interests in preparing for and in maintaining and supporting engagement in productive work in society	Home (work) life temporarily halted due to condition
4. Engage in clarification of goals and values in situations that demand personal involvement	Withdrawn from usual life situations at present
5. Act with responsibility in life situations in accordance with one's role or roles	Role diminished temporarily due to hospitalisation
6. Seek to understand the value of positive emotions	Sees positive emotions as valuable. 'You've got to laugh'
7. Seek to understand that negative emotions and action impulses are experienced when conduct is in discord with one's life goals and self-ideal	Understands that negative emotions are 'all part of life'
8. Promote positive mental health through deliberate efforts to function within a veridical (reality) frame of reference	Quite pragmatic and realistic about life
9. Function to bring about and maintain order in daily living	Order in living dictated by hospital routine at present
10. Function with integrity	Able to function with integrity
11. Function as a person in community	Not living in usual community at present; hospitalised
12. Function with increasing understanding of one's own humanity	Good understanding of her own humanity

Figure 3.4 Assessment of Mrs Butler's self-care deficits.

Source: Adapted from Orem, D.E. (2001) *Nursing: Concepts of Practice* (6th edn). London: Mosby.

Table 3.3 Care plan for Mrs Butler

Self-care deficit	Goal	Specific nursing actions	Description of general nursing actions	Review instructions (reduce as condition improves)
Preventing hazards to human life, human functioning and wellbeing	Treatment of hazard to human life (heart failure)	Administer pharmacological therapy as required/prescribed Intravenous/oral diuretic therapy Intravenous/oral nitrate therapy to keep systolic BP > 100mmHg ACE inhibitor	Providing physical support	Hourly
	Observe effectiveness of treatment	Evaluate effectiveness of diuretic and other pharmacological therapy	Providing physical support	Hourly
	Early detection of hazards to human life	Continuous ECG monitoring to detect life-threatening arrhythmias Observe for signs of worsening heart failure Preparation for and support during echocardiography investigations if required Management of arrhythmias Assess blood pressure and pulse rate Maintenance of patency and hygiene of intravenous line Monitoring and reporting electrolyte levels and administering treatment as prescribed	Providing physical support	Continuous evaluation through monitoring Hourly review of blood pressure
Maintaining a sufficient intake of air	To ensure optimum oxygen intake	Sit in upright position Administer oxygen Monitoring oxygen saturation continuously Monitor respiratory rate hourly Observe colour for signs of cyanosis Observe breathing pattern for regularity and signs of breathlessness Provide additional respiratory support if condition requires	Providing physical support	Review respiratory status hourly

	To reduce myocardial oxygen demand	Maintain on bed rest for at least 4 hours / Restrict activity in initial 24 hours	Guiding and directing	Review daily / Activity level may be increased slowly as condition improves
Maintaining a sufficient intake of water	To prevent fluid overload	Restrict fluid intake according to patient's condition observe urinary output hourly (1.5 litres/24 hours) / Monitor and record accurate fluid intake and output / Implement measures to maintain adequate fluid balance / Weigh daily to assess potential fluid retention	Providing physical support	Review hourly
Providing care associated with elimination processes and excrements	To provide assistance with elimination while activity is restricted	Provide assistance when using elimination facilities while activity is restricted / Provide assistance with hygiene needs while activity is restricted / Ensure patient dignity is maintained and appropriate level of self-care / Maintain hygiene of urinary catheter and ensure removal once appropriate	Acting for or doing for another	Review daily
Maintaining a balance between solitude and social interaction	To facilitate balance between solitude and social interaction while hospitalised	Facilitate visiting of family and provide family contacts as appropriate / Ensure that patient receives adequate periods of rest	Providing psychological support / Providing and maintaining an environment that supports personal development	Review daily
Human functioning and development within social groups	To acknowledge the temporary loss of normal social role and to provide support	Demonstrate empathy and understanding of Mrs Butler's feelings in this situation / Ensure maintenance of family contacts / Foster Mrs Butler's sense of self	Providing psychological support / Providing and maintaining an environment that supports personal development	Review daily
Being aware of and attending to the effects and results of pathological conditions and states	To ensure that the condition of myocardial infarction is understood upon discharge	Explanation of the anatomy and physiology of the heart / Explanation of pathology of heart failure / Explanation of causes and results of heart failure / Provide booklets and reading material to support information given	Teaching / Guiding and directing	Evaluate explanations daily / Review at discharge

Table 3.3 continued

Self-care deficit	Goal	Specific nursing actions	Description of general nursing actions	Review instructions (reduce as condition improves)
Effectively carrying out medically prescribed measures	To ensure that Mrs Butler understands medication requirements upon discharge	Explanation of the reason for medication being prescribed / Explanation of the medication action and effects / Explanation of timing, dosage and mode of administration of medication / Relevant teaching of medication administration if required / Explanation of the importance of taking medication on time / Explain potential side-effects of medication / Provide information on whom to contact if side effects to medication occur / Provide information of support available for management of medication (e.g. heart failure nurse)	Teaching / Guiding and directing	Evaluate explanations daily / Review at discharge
Learning to live with the effects of health state and treatment in a lifestyle that promotes continued personal development	To encourage and facilitate adoption of a lifestyle that will promote health and reduce recurrence of acute heart failure events	Clear and specific teaching and explanation about the importance of lifestyle modification / Strict adherence to medication regime / Using hospital supports to guide medication regime / Daily weights to assess level of fluid retention / Reporting signs of increased weight and or breathlessness immediately to healthcare provider to initiate prompt treatment / Avoiding foods that are high in salt content / Avoiding excessive alcohol intake / Provide information and contacts for relevant support groups / Provide information leaflets as appropriate / Referral to nurse-led clinic/cardiac rehabilitation		Evaluate explanations daily / Review at discharge

Adapted from Orem, D.E. (2001) Nursing: Concepts of Practice (6th edn). London, Mosby a debilitating condition, and it is essential to empower Mrs Butler to function according to her human potential and her desire to be normal. The teaching and supportive role in this case is crucial. Teaching focuses upon improving Mrs Butler's understanding of her condition and evaluating this understanding prior to discharge. It also aims to provide specific advice and direction with regard to prescribed medication that is essential for maintaining stability of the condition. Information and advice about lifestyle factors that affect or worsen heart failure, such as excessive alcohol intake, are given. Support and teaching continue after discharge where possible. Having a contact phone number where instant advice is available is valuable to patients like Mrs Butler and there are increasing numbers of nurse-led heart failure clinics offering specialist support and teaching to patients, including phone and home follow up in some cases. Where nurse-led initiatives are available, the nurse in CCU liaises with this service. Nurse-led services are discussed in more detail in Chapter 7.

Summary and conclusions

These case studies serve to illustrate conceptual model use based upon Orem's (2001) self-care deficit nursing theory. Although not definitive prescriptions for care, they provide some guidance for individualised care planning in the coronary care practice setting. These case studies of conceptual-model-based nursing highlight the complex and inclusive nature of the nursing assessment, planning intervention and evaluation. The notion of promoting self-care is evident in the care plans and helps to conceptualise patients as self-care agents, who wish to achieve their full potential in life. Considering patient care as a progression from wholly to partially compensatory and then to supportive highlights the ultimate aim of self-care. Using this model, education and teaching are viewed as pivotal to the nurse's role, and nursing actions in this area can be clearly identified and documented. As lifestyle management and correct use of prescribed medication is of great benefit in assisting many cardiac patients to achieve their full potential, this important nursing function is emphasised.

References

Connaughton, M. (2001) *Evidence Based Coronary Care*. London: Churchill Livingstone.

Department of Health (2000) *National Service Framework for Coronary Heart Disease*. London: Department of Health.

Gould, M. (2002) Chronic heart failure. In: Hatchett, R. and Thompson, D. (eds) *Cardiac Nursing*. London: Harcourt Publishing Ltd.

Hatchett, R. and Thompson, D. (2002) (eds) *Cardiac Nursing*. London: Harcourt Publishing Ltd.

ISIS-2 (1988) Second International Study of Infarct Survival Collaborate Group Randomised trial of intravenous streptokinase, oral aspirin, both or neither among 17,187 cases of suspected acute myocardial infarction. *Lancet* 345: 669–685.

Jowett, N.I. and Thompson, D.R. (2000) *Comprehensive Coronary Care*, 2nd edn. London: Baillière Tindall.

Meleis, A.I. (1997) *Theoretical Nursing Development and Progress*, 3rd edn. New York: Lippincott.

McMurray, J.J.V. and Stewart, S. (2001) The increasing burden of chronic heart failure. In: Stewart, S. and Blue, L. (eds) *Improving Outcomes in Chronic Heart Failure*. London: BMJ Books.

Norris, R.M. (1998) Fatality outside hospital from acute coronary events in three British Health Districts 1994–5. United Kingdom Heart Attack Study Collaborative Group. *British Medical Journal* 316: 1065–1070.

Orem, D.E. (1971, 1980, 1985, 1995, 2001) *Nursing: Concepts of Practice*, 1st, 2nd, 3rd, 4th 5th and 6th edns. London: Mosby.

Pearson, A., Vaughan, B. and Fitzgerald, M. (2001) *Nursing Models for Practice*. 2nd edn. London: Butterworth Heinemann.

Quinn, T., Webster, R. and Hatchett, R. (2002) Coronary heart disease: angina and acute myocardial infarction. In: Hatchett, R. and Thompson, D. (eds) *Cardiac Nursing*. London: Harcourt Publishing Ltd.

Quinn, T. (1999) Personal view. Thrombolysis in accident and emergency: the exception not the rule. Are we denying patients lifesaving treatment? *Accident and Emergency Nursing* 7(1): 39–41.

Sharpe, N. and Doughty, R. (1998) Epidemiology of heart failure and ventricular dysfunction. *Lancet* 352: 3–7.

Chapter 4

Role of the nurse in risk factor management

Key points
• Risk factor management is a priority for individuals with established CHD and high-risk individuals.
• Current approaches to risk factor management are inconsistent.
• Recent approaches to cardiac education have advocated needs-based programmes tailored to individual patient's needs.
• One additional dimension that has been recently added to the individualised approach is the use of behavior change models, notably the TTM (Prochaska and DiClemente 1982, 1984).
• The role of the nurse in risk factor management is still in developmental stages in many areas and it has been postulated that nurses are in an optimum position to lead a dedicated risk factor management services for CHD patients.

Risk factor management in the coronary care unit

Many patients who present to the coronary care unit (CCU) have underlying coronary heart disease (CHD). This is a broad term that refers to the effects of the atherosclerosis in the coronary arteries (De Backer et al. 2003). Patients presenting to CCU with acute coronary syndromes initially require nursing focusing on prevention of hazards to human life and maintaining sufficient intake of air. These actions involve providing physical support to individuals, which wholly or partially compensates for the individual's usual self-care. As the individual's condition improves and they gradually returns to self-care, nursing care augments recovery through supportive-educative actions. This involves teaching and guidance to raise the patient's awareness of the effects and results of his or her condition, to enable them to carry out medically prescribed measures and to adopt a lifestyle that promotes health.

The latter is an essential aspect of patient care in the CCU. Whether or not patients receive invasive treatment such as coronary artery bypass surgery or angioplasty, those individuals with CHD are predisposed to the development of angina or MI and are at a greater risk of sudden death. Thus there is a strong impetus to provide individuals with information that will assist them to reduce their risk of developing on-going disease (angina) or having life-threatening or fatal events (MI).

Risk factor management traditionally involved the provision of information and advice to patients about ways to reduce their risk of having another heart attack. Principal areas in which advice and intervention are given are diet, exercise and weight reduction, smoking cessation and taking of medications. This forms a component of a formalised concept of care delivery known as cardiac rehabilitation, aimed at restoring individuals to optimal health and preventing disease progression. Structured programmes have been in existence for more than 30 years. Traditionally, these programmes were concerned with the rehabilitation of those who had suffered acute MI, however, in many locations today, these services have been extended to all patients who are hospitalised with coronary artery diseases and not only those with MI.

What are risk factors?

CHD is the commonest cause of death in Europe, resulting in 2 million deaths each year (British Heart Foundation 2000). It accounts for 7.1 million deaths per year globally (World Health Organization 2003). It has been described by Quinn et al. 2002: 151) as 'the major cause of ill health and premature death in the developed world'. CHD accounts for 42% of all deaths from cardiovascular disease (CVD), which, it is estimated, will be the leading cause of death in developing countries by 2010 (World Health Organization 2003).

As both the morbidity and mortality from CHD disease are high in the Western world, much effort has been expended isolating the factors that contribute to the development of CHD, with a view to curtail its progress. Several risk factors have been identified that, when present in an individual, place them at a higher risk of developing the disease. An early-prospective study in the USA, known as the Framingham Study, contributed much to development of knowledge in this area and its results are widely reported.

The Framingham Study established clear links between elevated serum cholesterol, cigarette smoking and hypertension and the development of CHD (Daly-Nee et al. 1999). Daly-Nee et al. (1999) labelled these risk factors the 'classic triad'. In an overview of risk factors they provided detailed evidence supporting these risk factors and their contribution to the development of CHD. CHD is now considered to be 'strongly related to lifestyle' and risk factor modification has been 'unequivocally shown to reduce mortality and morbidity' (De Backer et al. 2003).

Other identified risk factors are diabetes, physical inactivity, obesity, low socioeconomic status, gender (more common in men) and heredity. Risk also increases with age. The classification of risk factors varies internationally. Some may be regarded as modifiable (high cholesterol, hypertension, cigarette smoking, physical inactivity, diabetes and obesity) or as non-modifiable (age, low socio-economic status, gender and heredity). The American Heart Association categorises these risk factors according to the magnitude of their effect and level of proof associated with risk: category I risk factors (the classic triad) having the greatest magnitude and where intervention has been *proven* to lower risk, while category IV risk factors have the least magnitude of effect and these refer to factors that cannot be modified (age, male gender, low socio-economic status and family history) (Daly-Nee et al. 1999).

Still other potential risk factors include alcohol consumption, described as having a 'complex interplay between consumption and risk' (Rippe and O'Brien 1999: 47).

Moderate amounts appear to reduce risk in several studies, however, heavier alcohol consumption appears to increase risk. Elevated homocysteine levels also place an individual at increased risk and Rippe and O'Brien (1999) cite recent studies which suggest that the intake of daily folate may reduce homocysteine levels.

Patients who develop CHD often attribute this development to stress. However, the evidence base to support this is not convincing and further research needs to be done in this area. Older studies and texts indicated that personality type was a contributory factor, however, Rippe and O'Brien (1999) indicated that this latter area, and stress in general, remain 'controversial' as definitive risk factors.

The value of formalised *primary* prevention initiatives, with community screening for CHD and risk factor management for individuals without recognised CHD has not been clearly established. A Cochrane review (Ebrahim and Davey Smith 2001) suggested that primary interventions are of limited benefit in the general population. There is little evidence to support the benefits of primary healthcare interventions, other than to individuals identified as high risk (Daly-Nee et al. 1999).

Secondary prevention aims to slow down disease progression and reduce mortality in those individuals who have confirmed CHD. The modification and control of risk factors improves outcomes and an individual's 'risk' may be reduced. In this case, it is not the risk of *developing* CHD, but rather of worsening of the disease.

'Patients with established cardiovascular disease have declared themselves to be at high risk of a further vascular event. Therefore, they require the most intensive lifestyle intervention' (De Backer et al. 2003). This may seem an anomaly, that prevention is targeted at those who already have the disease, rather than those without. However, active risk factor management in this population has an estimated reduction 'of about a third in coronary morbidity and mortality with corresponding increase in life expectancy' (Wood 1998). Therefore, an active commitment to risk factor management in all patients with CHD could really add years to life and life to years.

Risk may be described as 10-year absolute risk of developing a fatal event (Pyoräla et al. 1994, De Backer et al. 2003). This event may be a CHD event (Pyoräla et al. 1994), however, it is important to recognise that this risk also pertains to cardiovascular events in general (De Backer et al. 2003).

At present secondary prevention is the mainstay of nursing intervention in the CCU, patients presenting to the coronary care nurse usually have CHD and can benefit from risk management advice. This is an important aspect of the nursing role as nurses are confronted, daily, with a priority group requiring risk factor management. Nurse-led initiatives in this area have much to offer with regard to long-term outcome.

Active risk factor management occurs on a number of levels. First, identifying risk factors in individuals during an assessment procedure, and secondly, delivering an effective formalised system that results in risk factor modification. However, in reality, the process is not that simple for a variety of reasons.

Challenges to risk factor management in the practice setting

Risk factor management reflects a formalised relationship between individuals and health professionals that actively engages them in risk factor reduction. Recent advice on risk factor management supports the use of a formalised system that identifies risks in patients with CHD or high-risk individuals and targets them appropriately. The system needs to have on-going support beyond discharge and have a mechanism for giving and receiving feedback.

This system should also be able to cater for assessment and management of multiple risk factors, rather than dealing with one in isolation. Purely focusing on one risk factor, such as smoking, although valid, leads to fragmenting of the risk management and prioritises certain aspects of behaviour, which may be inappropriate. Risk factors tend to 'cluster' in individuals (Grundy et al. 1998), placing them at a higher overall risk. Contemporary practice highlights the need to consider the multiplicity of risk factors present and the increased negative impact that this has on risk (Pyoräla et al. 1994, De Backer et al. 2003).

There is no agreed format for risk factor management. The interventions vary. Ad hoc advice and information are often given to patients, either verbally or written down, by nursing and medical staff in the hospital setting. In the past, concern with informal information giving encouraged formalised education programmes for cardiac patients. The level of provision of these is unclear, and it is common to find formalised education programmes as components of cardiac rehabilitation.

From a worldwide perspective, not all hospitals provide this service. Horgan et al. noted in 1992 that less than half the hospitals in the UK and Ireland had cardiac rehabilitation services. Although Horgan et al. (1992) recommended that all hospitals should provide this service, the level of service is not consistent between hospitals nationally or internationally, and it is unlikely that all patients receive formalised lifestyle advice. Indeed, Gambling (2003) noted in her study in the UK that patients with CHD felt a sense of 'lack of direction or focus [and] bewilderment' after discharge. Many of them reported receiving little advice on lifestyle. While this lack of information may pertain to patient retention, it also highlights that patients may have received the information/advice informally and in many cases patients do not have adequate resources after discharge.

There is, however, some evidence to suggest that gaps exist in the provision of risk factor advice in the hospital setting. De Backer et al. (2003) noted the reality of risk factor management in the practice setting falls well below expectations suggesting 'a serious gap between recommendations . . . and the advice actually provided by physicians in routine clinical practice'. Wood (1998) also noted that this 'progress is slow in the integration of coronary heart disease prevention into daily clinical practice by cardiologists and other physicians . . .'.

A similar picture emerges in the community setting. Bowker et al. (1996) concluded from a national survey of coronary patients in the UK that both management and recording of risk factors were 'less than optimal'. Although information regarding the presence of potential risk factors was available for over 70% of patients this was more likely for those undergoing invasive procedures such as bypass surgery or coronary angiography Cholesterol measurements were available for only less than half of the patients.

Specific actions related to risk factor management were inconsistently reported. The most frequently cited response was actions for hypertension (at least 60% of cases). Smoking and weight advice/intervention was noted infrequently (no action recorded for at least 50% of cases). Cholesterol action was recorded in almost 50% of cases.

This study clearly indicates that gaps exist in current provision. While health professionals in both the community and hospital setting have ample opportunity to record and possibly advise on risk factor management, opportunities are missed possibly due to lack of formalised structures and time and resource constraints.

International literature on this area is scarce and many opportunities are likely to be missed in the practice setting, possibly due to the pragmatic need to prioritise on the patient's presenting problem. This focus on the main presenting medical problem, such as hypertension in Bowker et al. (1996), while necessary and important, leaves a gap in relation to the multiplicity of risk factors and the importance of their control in disease management. The value of simultaneously addressing all risk factors cannot be ignored.

The way forward appears to be an active risk management programme that deals exclusively with empowering individuals to manage their risk factors operating within the community or local hospital setting. This may involve support and advice on a diet that is low in saturated fat, weight reduction, exercise, smoking cessation, alcohol moderation and compliance to prescribed medication for hypertension and raised cholesterol. This needs to be tailored to individual needs. Lancaster and Steed (2001) in a Cochrane review noted that there was evidence to suggest that tailoring programmes to suit individual needs is more effective.

Other factors known to contribute to success are facilitation, reinforcement, and feedback (Mullen et al. 1992). These factors open to us the possibility that the intervention should not only be individualised but also *personalised*. It is perhaps insufficient to consider only teaching/learning methodologies. We need to engage with the patient in a way that encourages change and we also need to develop an understanding of the complexities of initiating and maintaining change.

Recent approaches to achieving sustained behavioural changes in risk factors (exercise increase, dietary changes, weight loss, smoking cessation and compliance) have begun to examine the *stage* of change that the individual is in at the time of assessment, and provide responsive, supportive information. This upturns the traditional notion of patient education as merely information giving. Rather than imparting something to the patient (information/education) in the hope it will be effective, it meets the patient half way, by finding out where the patient is at in terms of his or her own necessary changes. Although this is, in a sense, identifying patient needs, it goes a little further than that by actually finding out whether or not the individual is responsive to change at this time and providing interventions appropriate to each stage.

This requires planning interventions based on a model that clearly explains the behaviour change process. One popular behaviour change model is the transtheoretical model (TTM) (Prochaska and DiClemente 1982, 1984). From examining the behaviours of thousands of people, Prochaska and DiClemente noted that individuals may be considered to be in one of five stages of change at any one time, and that processes of change facilitate success at various stages.

A behaviour change model: transtheoretical model

The stages and processes of the TTM (Prochaska and DiClemente 1982, 1984) have achieved validity and reliability from years of empirical study, and have recently been mooted as extremely promising for risk factor management in cardiac patients.

Rossi and Rossi (1999) have been very optimistic about the potential contribution of the TTM to behaviour change in CHD. They suggested that it could help to understand, explain, and reduce CHD risk. 'The TTM is particularly relevant because it is rapidly emerging as one of the most promising models applied to multiple risk-factor reduction' (Rossi and Rossi 1999: 57). It is interesting to note that the TTM has also been applied effectively to adopting *new* behaviours (exercise), and not only to cessation of addictive behaviours (Nigg and Riebe 2002).

Prochaska et al. (1994) described how they spent several years studying the ways that people intentionally change. They searched for an underlying structure of change that is common to both self-change and intervention-led change. They examined whether basic principles of change existed and they suggested that there is quite compelling evidence that they do.

They described the development of their model over a series of more than 50 studies on thousands of individuals examining how people overcome issues such as smoking, alcohol abuse, weight control, emotional distress and others. They uncovered 'a revolution in the science of behaviour change' (Prochaska et al. 1994: 14) which precipitated a paradigm shift in the way that behaviours are dealt with in the clinical setting.

From their interviews with successful self-changers it emerged that change followed a series of stages described as: pre-contemplation, contemplation, preparation, action and maintenance. Individuals 'typically recycle through these stages several times before termination of the addiction' (Prochaska et al. 1992). Following an assessment, individuals may be categorised into one of these five stages. The value of this is that the approach can be modified according to the stage.

Individuals in the pre-contemplation stage, for example do not want to change. Intensive intervention may not be appropriate, although brief information and resources may be provided. Those in the contemplation stage are beginning to think about the possibility of change. They are open to suggestion and may be responsive to intervention. Those in the preparation stage are actively pre-empting action and require support. Those in action stage have begun their commitment, and require specific support. Those in maintenance have taken on the new behaviour and require on-going support.

Prochaska et al. (1992) described the stages of change as a spiral model as people often do not proceed neatly from one stage to the next. They may regress and go back and forth several times before success. They noted that their research indicates that many people who relapse regress to contemplation or preparation rather than pre-contemplation, so even though they may feel a failure they are still further along than at first.

When discussing the treatment implications of this model Prochaska et al. noted that the usual education/intervention programmes are 'action orientated' and are likely to fail, as 'the vast majority of [addicted] people are *not* in the action stage'. Across many studies, they suggested, up to 60% of people are in the precontemplation stage with only 10–15% prepared for action. This is surprisingly few people who are openly responsive to change, and warrants an understanding of the correct actions required for those in the pre-action stages.

Thompson (1999) suggested that those working in cardiac rehabilitation programmes would benefit from developing an understanding of how people change.

She suggested focusing nursing action on contemplators and preparers because 'the pre-contemplators are not ready to change and the actors and maintainers are managing'. She suggested that the stages of change model 'theoretically holds great promise'.

Understanding an individual's willingness or readiness to change is pivotal to the operation of the TTM. 'Probably the most obvious and direct implication of our research is the need to assess the stage of a client's readiness for change and to tailor interventions accordingly' (Prochaska et al. 1994: 75). They suggested that although clinicians may do this instinctively, they found little evidence for this in the research. 'We have determined that efficient self-change depends on doing the right things (processes) at the right time (stages)' (Prochaska et al. 1994: 75). They reinforced that intervention needs to be matched to the stage of change and suggested that traditional programmes were action orientated, while beneficial to those in the action stage but 'ineffective or detrimental' to those in pre-contemplation or contemplation stages. This is substantial, given that their research indicated that the vast majority of people fall into the pre-contemplation stage. They suggested many US programmes across healthcare settings are 'mismatched'.

The literature on the use of TTM presents several distinct aspects of the use of this model in practice. First, the development and description of the stages of change are well documented. The assessment procedure is commonly referred to and relates specifically to how the stages of change are identified. Secondly, the provision of support and intervention focus on the *processes* of change identified by Prochaska and DiClemente (1982, 1984). These are conciousness raising, self-re-evaluation, social re-evaluation, self-liberation, social liberation, counter-conditioning, stimulus control, contingency management, dramatic relief and helping relationship.

Much of the literature on the management of risk factors positively endorses use of the TTM providing evidence of effectiveness of interventions. Much has been written about the important role of self-efficacy (confidence) in the change process.

Stages of change

Prochaska et al. (1994) have described *pre-contemplation* as a stage of denial and an active resistance to change; how individuals are often stuck in this phase and question 'whether help is even a possibility' (1994: 75). These individuals often give up on change, and give up on themselves.

Those in the phase of pre-contemplation use defences to explain their behaviour including denial, minimising behaviour and providing plausible excuses for behaviour (rationalisation). They may also turn their feelings outward using projection and displacement, accusing others of having the behaviour. They have no intention to change in the near future. Sometimes individuals 'just don't see the problem' (Prochaska et al. 1994).

Contemplation is the stage where individuals are considering change, but may not be quite ready to start. It is symbolised by an awareness of the problem, however, people can also become stuck in this stage. Prochaska et al. (1994) have described a state of 'chronic contemplation'. These individuals say they will change someday. They desire change but simultaneously resist it. It often involves 'the search for absolute certainty', with some individuals carefully scrutinising the facts but never taking action. They may display signs of 'waiting for the magic moment' or 'wishful thinking' to solve their problems.

Individuals in the *preparation* stage of change intend to act on their problem in the immediate future. This stage of change is characterised by small steps toward action, such as reducing the number of cigarettes smoked per day. Preparation is also characterised by recent unsuccessful attempts at behaviour change. It is this combination of intention to change with a behavioural pattern of recent attempts to change that distinguishes individuals in the preparation stage from those in contemplation.

The *action* stage is a period of active en-gagement in changing the problem behaviour and is what most people, including clinicians, think of as behaviour change. The period of action is usually described as lasting for 6 months, as this typically encompasses the period of greatest risk of relapse for many problem behaviours. To reach the action stage individuals must meet strict criteria of behaviour change, such as quitting smoking, losing a specified amount of weight, reducing dietary fat or exercising on a regular basis. *Maintenance* stage is when the individual has sustained the behaviour change for at least 6 months.

It is helpful, from the perspective of a practising nurse, to know what stage of change an individual may be in, and use this to guide risk factor intervention.

Assessing the stage of change

There is agreement in the research literature that use of the TTM model in practice requires assessment of the stages of change to support health behaviour change interventions (Buxton et al. 1996). Burkholder and Evers (2002) concluded that the *stages of change* framework is a valid and reliable way of assessing the position of individuals with regard to behaviour change in this area.

Prochaska et al. (1994) recommended that the assessment of the stage of change should be a straightforward process. They suggest presenting four simple statements to the patients to ascertain a level of agreement with each statement (yes or no) (Box 4.1).

The response is used to indicate the individual's purported stage of change. Those who are in the pre-contemplation stage usually answer 'no' to all statements. Contemplators answer 'yes' to statement four and 'no' to all the others. Those in the preparation stage say 'yes' to statement three and four and 'no' to all the others. In the action stage individuals say 'yes' to statement two and 'no' to statement one.

Box 4.1 Assessment of stage of change

I solved my problem more than 6 months ago	yes/no
I have taken action on my problem within the past 6 months	yes/no
I am intending to take action in the next month	yes/no
I am intending to take action in the next 6 months	yes/no

Adapted from Prochaska et al. (1994) *Changing for Good. The Revolutionary Program that Explains the Six Stages of Change and Teaches You How to Free Yourself from Bad Habits.* New York: William Morrow and Co.

When an individual can answer 'yes' truthfully to statement one they have achieved maintenance stage (Prochaska et al. 1994).

Another method for assessing a patient's stage of change was proposed by Houston Miller and Taylor (1995), who suggested that the assessment might be simply done by asking a patient if he or she intends to undertake a particular action. They may be asked then to rate their intention of adopting behaviour on a scale of zero to eight (zero indicating no intention, eight indicating absolute intention). They found this model useful in practice and in their experience those who indicated little or no intention to change were unlikely to do so. Thus in practice they focus more on individuals who have expressed a desire to change. It is unclear whether or not this method is sensitive enough to identify stages of change other than those in pre-contemplation (who do not want to change), although Houston Miller and Taylor reported successful use.

Another way of assessing stage of change in the literature is the use of an open style interview that allows the patient to freely express their views. This is in direct contrast to many assessment procedures that are documentation based and are carried out in time-confined schedules. This notion of allowing a reasonable time for interview is favourable to patients. The practice nurses in Wiles' study in 1994 carried out very short secondary prevention interviews due to time constraints, and it subsequently emerged that the patients would have liked more time.

Priest and Speller (1991: 15) support the use of the open style interview for risk general risk factor screening based on the stages of change model, which they term 'motivational interview'. The goal of the interview is to 'lead the patient to talk as much as possible about why he feels he should change'.

Williams also advocates the interview approach suggesting a 'focused interview' using open-ended questions to assess stages of change. She suggested that 'nurses play a key role in assessing the risk factors that lead to disease expression and in intervening to help individuals modify risk behaviours' (1999: 72). Similarly, Kristeller (1999) suggested the use of a patient-centred counselling approach with use of open questioning to assess the stages of change for the management of smoking as a risk factor in cardiac disease. She suggests the first question to ask when assessing motivation is 'How do you feel about your smoking [behaviour]?' followed by 'How do you feel about stopping [behaviour]?' (Kristeller 1999: 73). A good question for the pre-contemplator is 'What do you like about smoking [behaviour]?'

The use of patient interviews is not necessarily a new phenomenon for CCU nurses, who spend quite a considerable amount of time closely assessing patients and collecting patient information. It is of course a challenge in units when time and resources are limited. However, the benefit with this suggested mode of practice is eliciting information on whether or not patients are willing to change behaviour. Using this approach may deem that some patients are not ready to receive information (pre-contemplators) and resources saved by providing limited information to these individuals, may actually allow more time for interviews to take place. A more time wise approach is Prochaska et al.'s (1994) suggestion of a simple straight-forward assessment process (see Box 4.1), a useful instrument that can be easily applied in the clinical setting. It is useful to explore areas of practice where this approach has been used successfully.

The practice experience

Assessment of stages of change has been successfully in practice. Jue and Cunningham (1998) successfully assessed and described the stages of change regarding adoption of exercise by patients following coronary artery bypass surgery using a
self-reporting questionnaire between 4–6 and 22–26 months after hospital discharge. The majority of patients were in the maintenance stage (67%) and had been
exercising for more than 6 months. Seven per cent were in pre-contemplation, 11%
in contemplation, 5% in preparation and 10% in action.

Loughlan and Mutrie (1997) used the ability to identify the stages of change to
select a sample of hospital staff that they believed were open to change. Those
candidates who were deemed to be either in the contemplation or in the preparation
phase only were randomly assigned to lifestyle intervention groups, with positive
results. Hilton et al. (1999) allocated patients from GP practices after assessment to
one of the five stages of change for each of their cardiac lifestyle behaviours (pre-
contemplation, contemplation, preparation, action and maintenance). They re-
assessed at 4 months and then at 12 months. They were confident that this approach
had potential in the GP setting. Rather than opting for a 'blanket approach' this
method of assessment elucidates 'the most effective means of targeting and managing those with existing disease, or those at high risk of developing it' (Hilton et al.
1999).

Similarly, Finckenor and Byrd-Bredbenner (2000) noted that candidates in either
pre-contemplation, contemplation or preparation stages made significant changes
upon intervention compared with those in the 'action/maintenance stage (as they
had already initiated changes). They suggested that grouping individuals at similar
stages together might be effective. Hall Sims and Zucker (1999) used an assessment
of stages of change to underpin a nursing intervention for smoking cessation. For
pre-contemplators, where the smoker had not decided to stop, they found it is useful
to distribution self-help material and self-monitoring techniques such as record
keeping. They also made a follow-up phone call after 1 week. Contemplators were
advised to stop smoking, provided self-help material and discussed tapering cigarettes and the use of nicotine replacement therapy. In the action stage the nurse discussed what the smoker has tried in the past to determine what was unsuccessful in
previous attempts.

These studies clearly illustrate that the stages of change (TTM) can be used in a
variety of ways to clearly categorise individuals within various client groups and this
serves practice in a useful way. The studies identified innovative ways of employing
the assessment findings, such as tailored intervention which is stage dependent; provision of basic information to those in pre-contemplation, so that they have the
necessary resources should they progress to the contemplation phase; and grouping
individuals according to stage of change category for teaching purposes. This latter
suggestion by Finckenor and Byrd-Bredbenner (2000) has useful implications for
cost savings in this area.

Jordan and Nigg (2002) highlighted that assessing the initial stage of change that
a person is in with subsequent tailoring of interventions yielded positive outcomes in
several studies. While individualisation of assessment heralds cost implications, this
does not require dismissal of this notion. Rather, innovative strategies such as web-

based assessment or grouping of individuals from similar categories requires consideration.

Once the stage of change has been identified the appropriate intervention needs to be implemented.

Support and intervention – processes of change

The literature indicates that focus should be placed on those who are responsive to treatment and actually want to change, effectively all persons, except those deemed to be in the pre-contemplation stage. However, this raises ethical implications for healthcare, and this area requires further research and development.

Programmes based on the stages of change involve the usual risk factor management education and advice with an added dimension known as the *processes* of change (Prochaska and DiClemente 1984). These processes are known to occur in individuals during their change and include: consciousness raising, self-re-evaluation, social re-evaluation, self-liberation, social liberation, counter-conditioning, stimulus control, contingency management, dramatic relief and helping relationship. All these processes have been found to assist individuals in making change a reality. They are used across the five stages, and use of each one depends on particular stage. Knowledge of the interaction between processes and stages helps the nurse to use the process as an intervention, and support these processes in individuals. Prochaska and DiClemente (1984) have described how these five stages of change integrate with the processes.

Burkholder and Evers (2002) concluded that the processes of change were valid and consistently related to the stages of change. The pre-contemplation stage uses the least change processes. Respondents in this stage in Prochaska and DiClemente's study (1983) used eight out of ten of the processes, which was significantly less than the other subjects. Consciousness raising was a common feature of the contemplation stage, with self-re-evaluation bridging both the contemplation and the action stage. Self-liberation emerged when individuals took action. Helping relationship, reinforcement and management also emerged here. Counter-conditioning and stimulus control bridged both action and maintenance and these processes were emphasised during both phases.

Prochaska et al. (1994) described how the knowledge of the relationship between processes and stages can helps successful intervention. For pre-contemplators, consciousness raising (raising awareness) and developing a solid helping relationship is useful. The nurse should try to develop a supporting relationship with the patient and alert him or her to the potential outcomes of the behaviour(s) in question (to raise consciousness about the implications). Prochaska et al. (1994) suggest that this should avoid pushing the person into action. 'A pre-contemplator is not ready to take action, but may be ready to consider changing' (Prochaska et al. 1994: 96). They suggest that acting as a helper involves objectively addressing specific behaviours and frequently recommend behaviour change rather than scolding or enabling the behaviour (avoiding discussions and confrontations, soften consequences by minimising events, make excuses, cover for and defend problem behaviours, indirectly or rarely recommend behaviour change).

Prochaska et al. (1994) suggest that contemplators even with awareness would not initiate action until they achieve a greater understanding of their behaviour. Consciousness raising is important at this stage. It is important that at this stage the nurse focuses on clearly alerting the patient to the potential outcomes of the behaviour(s) in question (to raise consciousness about the implications). Social liberation is also important. Perception that the avoidance of the behaviour may cause social isolation, or cause temptation acts as a barrier to change. It is useful therefore to assist individuals with creating more choice and alternatives for living/socialising, providing more information about problem behaviours and guidance towards public support venues for those who want to change (non-smoking areas/self-help groups). Changing lifestyle may require significant changes in social habits, and the individual may require quite basic support and advice with regard to this. As social liberation is a process, the individual who is successful in change will develop an awareness of the necessary social changes required.

Successful self-changers have reported that they valued helping relationships most during the stages of contemplation, preparation and action. Two techniques in particular were important for this empathy and warmth. Preparation takes a person from the decisions made in the contemplation stage to the specific steps taken to solve the problem during the action stage. At the outset of the research Prochaska et al. did not separate preparation from contemplation but it became evident that the differences are subtle. Their experience indicated that proper preparation is key to successful self-change. Rather than gathering information on the problem as in contemplation, this phase gathers information on possible actions (Prochaska et al. 1994).

Countering is useful in the action stage. This technique finds alternatives to problem behaviours such as an active diversion, exercise, relaxation or environmental control and reward. A patient could be encouraged to go for a walk for example, or exercise to counter the temptation to smoke. Discussion and support may elicit an activity that is most suited to the individual. The important point is to support the individual to avoid temptations appropriately and become aware of the need to do so.

In Jue and Cunningham's (1998) study in cardiac patients following coronary artery bypass surgery these processes were used during various stages of change. The subjects in the pre-contemplation and contemplation stages used the least number of change processes. The contemplators and the actors used the most. Counter-conditioning was used most frequently by maintainers.

Self-efficacy

Self-efficacy (confidence) has also been recognised as having an important role in changing behaviours, particularly in the maintenance stage (Prochaska and DiClemente 1982). Drawing on the work of Bandura (1977, 1982) Prochaska and DiClemente conceptualised self-efficacy as an individual's evaluation of their own ability to perform a task. They also suggested that self-efficacy contributed to self-liberation. Similarly, Jordan and Nigg (2002) highlighted how the concept of self-efficacy can be integrated usefully into the stages of change model and was found to be an important predictor of intermediate outcome and success.

Rossi and Rossi (1999) perceived this to be of particular relevance in risk factor reduction and referred to it as the 'confidence an individual has in his or her own ability to successfully carry out a particular behavior'. In practice, Houston Miller and Taylor (1995) found that measuring self-efficacy was useful for predicting success of cardiac risk factor behavioural interventions. They found that patient's ability to modify their behaviour, for example in the area of exercise was strongly influenced by their confidence. So rather than questioning patients about their ability, they suggested that the more prudent approach is to ask them about their confidence, which then may also be improved. Exercise as an activity was found to increase confidence (Ewart et al. 1983).

Using the self-efficacy construct within the TTM has typically taken the form of asking respondents how *confident* they are that they would not engage in a particular behaviour in difficult situations. Within the TTM, self-efficacy is assessed in two parts: confidence and temptation. Confidence is related to an individual's ability to deal with high-risk situations without engaging in specific behaviour and temptation is an individual's rating of the strength of his or her desire to engage in behaviours during high-risk situations. There is a strong relation between temptation and stage of change, with a linear decrease from pre-contemplation to maintenance (DiClemente et al. 1991, Prochaska et al. 1992).

Although temptation and confidence are related to one another, they do not necessarily overlap or operate in a simultaneous fashion. For smoking cessation, confidence scores peaked after about 18 months of prolonged abstinence (Rossi et al. 1999). Temptation scores, on the other hand, continued to decrease for up to 5 years after cessation. These results suggested that temptation might be a more sensitive measure of relapse potential than confidence and those even individuals who have been in the maintenance stage for several years are not completely free of risk. Confidence improves, however temptation is elusive and persistent.

Burkholder and Evers (2002) observed that the TTM has been used successfully in risk factor management. They revealed that self-efficacy was found to increase steadily across the stages of change, and this relation was supported in several studies. Clearly, ascertaining patients confidence level at the outset as well as supporting confidence development is an essential element that has hitherto eluded many health professionals as an intervention approach.

While there is consistent evidence that a multi-disciplinary approach to risk factor management is good practice, there is increasing recognition of the value of the nurse as central co-ordinator of team interventions. The use of the TTM model certainly creates an opportunity for nurses taking the lead in this area. The holistic approach used is congruent with nurses' supportive-educative actions. Furthermore, while specialist skills such as those of a physician, dietician and psychologist may be required in the process, the assessment, planning and co-ordinating of interventions is also consistent with nursing actions.

This approach was used successfully by Houston Miller and Taylor (1995) in the USA, whose nurse managed multi-disciplinary approach to cardiac risk factor management and rehabilitation yielded positive outcomes, and research that contributed significantly to our knowledge in this area. This work provides a useful template for those nurses considering developing their role in this way.

Developing the role of the nurse in risk factor management

The nurse's role in risk factor management (secondary prevention) has not been clearly articulated in the literature. Along with other health professionals nurses provide ad hoc information and advice, and some partake in formalised cardiac rehabilitation sessions. In some areas, practice nurses are actively involved in the provision of lifestyle advice to patients. However, given the expanding roles of nurses within many areas of cardiology, and the emergence and success of nurse-led care in many areas, there is certainly potential to develop specialist nurse roles within this area. In addition, formalising risk factor management with a dedicated nurse-led component in a variety of settings may also deal with the many missed opportunities for risk factor interventions in practice.

Fullard (1990) and Houston Miller and Taylor (1995) highlighted the key role that hospitals-based and practice-based nurses can play in risk factor management to reduce cardiovascular risk. For this to become a reality there are clear guidelines on workload, patient criteria, training and audit (Fullard, 1990). Fullard (1990) highlighted that an organised system of referral needs to be set up with clear indications for selection of patients.

Wiles (1994) identified practice (lifestyle) nurses as a good source of lifestyle advice for prevention of CHD. In Wiles' survey 85% of nurses reported delivering lifestyle advice to patients with CHD and 88% reported that they followed up some people regarding lifestyle advice. Interviews with 26 patients revealed that lifestyle advice was commonly given during routine visits to the practice. This occurred when patients, such self-referred for health checks/dietary advice and also opportunistically when patients were seen for something unrelated to lifestyle. Highlighting the potential contribution of practice nurses in risk management, Wiley recommended training in negotiating behaviour change to support their role.

The nurse intervention in the GP setting discussed above involved risk factor management for those with established disease. The potential value of the nurse role in this area is highlighted by the initiative demonstrated when the nurses opportunistically gave advice. This role of the nurse in GP settings could also be expanded to include risk factor intervention for individuals deemed to be at high risk. An individual referred to the service may have elevated serum cholesterol and may be a smoker. This individual although they may not have obvious CHD, is at a higher risk of developing the disease. The nurse can provide risk factor management advice, based on the individual's stage of change.

One recent development that may greatly enhance the work of the nurse in this area is De Backer et al.'s (2003) risk factor chart SCORE, which allows estimation of an individual's (without known disease) 10-year risk of having a fatal CVD event. For those individuals identified as contemplators or in preparation, this tool could serve to graphically and visually raise consciousness by highlighting the individual's risk of death using a scientifically derived tool.

The risk factors taken into account within this system are hypertension, raised serum cholesterol, age, gender and smoking status. It is a very useful tool for use in primary prevention settings, as it allows individuals to examine, visually, the influence that these risk factors have on their overall risk, and the net reduction on risk if the factor is modified (European Society of Cardiology 2004). It also takes into account regional variations within Europe, with an individual chart for low- and high-risk regions of Europe. It can also be adapted to suit particular populations or groups.

Patients in CCU, with established CHD, are not the target audience for the SCORE chart, as De Backer et al. have clearly stated that this group is *already* a high-risk category. Nurse risk factor interventions should still reflect a systematic approach to practice. All patients with CHD should receive appropriate risk factor advice and education. This should focus on control and modification of all known modifiable risks, such as raised serum cholesterol, hypertension, smoking, and lack of exercise. Where possible the approach should be personalised and tailored to individual needs. This complies with Orem's (2001) supportive-educative actions and involves teaching and guidance to raise the patient's awareness of the effects and results of their condition, enabling the patient to carry out medically prescribed measures and supporting the patient to learn to live in a lifestyle that promotes health.

Modifying risk factors often involve specific changes in lifestyle behaviour (e.g. taking medication, losing weight, modifying diet). Behaviour change is complex and specific education strategies are discussed in Chapter 5. Determining the individual's stage of change is a useful starting point as suggested in this chapter. Using a check-list or interview approach the nurse in CCU can easily determine whether or not the patient is likely to be responsive to the risk factor education. Houston Miller and Taylor (1995), pioneers of nurse-led cardiac rehabilitation intervention in the USA, suggest using the assessment strategy to focus the interventions on those who are ready to change.

Summary and conclusions

Recent approaches to education for cardiac patients have advocated needs-based programmes tailored to the individual patient's needs. This is considered to promote the programme success, rather than blanket information/education approaches. One dimension that has been recently added to the individualised approach is the use of behaviour change models, notably the TTM (Prochaska and DiClemente 1982, 1984) which clearly identifies the stages and processes of adult change behaviour. This guides clinicians to carefully assess patients' readiness to change and apply support according to their professed stage of change.

The TTM requires identification of individual's stage of change and individu-alised support of natural change processes. This has obvious resources implications, however, web-based systems can be developed to allow patients home access to at least some of the resource material. This innovation, together with Finckenor and Byrd-Bredbenner's (2000) suggestion of grouping together individuals at similar stages may be manageable alternatives that could reduce costs. These systems could be used in addition to some individual sessions, and perhaps phone-based support systems. It may be timely to centralise and standardise these systems of intervention. Phone support could be provided across a wide range of areas, if the adequate support systems were in place (such as computerised patient records). The integra-tion of this model of practice into current systems of care requires careful thought and planning by practitioners. Assessment of stages of change, which is the initial phase of the process, might be performed as part of a nursing assessment upon admission to a CCU and processes of support integrated into care planning (Chapter 3). Information of stages of change and intervention should then be communicated to relevant healthcare staff who will continue the education after discharge from the CCU (cardiac rehabilitation or other nurse-led services). Appropriate documentation and transfer of information to relevant personnel is essential.

The role of the nurse in risk factor management is still in the developmental stage in many areas and it has been postulated that nurses are in an optimum position to lead a dedicated risk factor management service for patients with CHD. The development of this role requires careful planning and should include specific training on lifestyle management to include an understanding of the TTM model.

The nursing profession acknowledges the need for continuous professional advancement in order to meet ever changing healthcare needs (Robinson 1991). In order to make a serious commitment to risk factor management nurses need to take the lead in planning, developing and managing interventions. The future is a 'kaleidoscope of new and infinite probability' (Hein 1998: 401).

References

Bandura A. (1977) *Social Learning Theory*. New Jersey: Prentice Hall.

Bandura A. (1982) Self-efficacy mechanism in human agency. *American Psychologist* 37: 122–147.

Bowker, T.J., Clayton, T.C., Pyke, D.M. and Wood, D.A. (1996) A British Cardiac Society survey of the potential for the secondary prevention of coronary disease: ASPIRE (Action on Secondary Prevention through Intervention to Reduce Events). *Heart* 75: 334–342.

British Heart Foundation (2000) *European Cardiovascular Disease Statistics*. London: British Heart Foundation.

Burkholder, G.J. and Evers, K. (2002) Application of the transtheoretical model to several problem behaviors. In: Burbank, P.M. and Riebe, D. (eds) *Promoting Exercise and Behavior Change in Older Adults: Interventions With the Transtheoretical Model*. New York: Springer Publishing Company.

Buxton, K., Wyse, J. and Mercer, T. (1996) How applicable is the *stages of change* model to exercise behaviour? A review. *Health Education Journal* 55: 239–257.

Daly-Nee C., Brunt, H. and Jairath, N. (1999) Risk and coronary heart disease. In: Jairath, N. (ed) *Coronary Heart Disease & Risk Factor Management: A Nursing Perspective*. London: W.B. Saunders.

De Backer, G., Ambrosioni, E., Borch-Johnsen, K., Brotons, C., Cifkova, R., Dallongeville, J., Ebrahim, S., Faergeman, O., Graham, I., Mancia, G., Manger Cats, V., Orth-Gomér, K., Perk, J., Pyörälä, K., Rodicio, J.L., Sans, S., Sansoy, V., Sechtem, U., Silber, S., Thomsen, T., and Wood, D. (2003) European guidelines on cardiovascular disease prevention in clinical practice. *European Heart Journal* 24: 1601–1610.

DiClemente, CC., Prochaska, J.Q., Vairhurst. S.K., Velicer, W.V., Velasquez, M.M., and Rossi, J.S. (1991) The process of smoking cessation: An analysis of precontemplation, contemplation arid preparation stages of change. *Journal of Consulting and Clinical Psychology* 59: 295–304.

Ebrahim, S. and Davey Smith, G. (2001) Multiple risk factor intervention for primary prevention of coronary heart disease. In: *Cochrane Library*. Issue 1, Oxford: Update Software.

European Society of Cardiology (2004) SCORE Chart Online. Available at www.escardio.org/initiatives/prevention/HeartScore.htm (accessed 13 April, 2004)

Ewart, C.K., Taylor, C.B., Reese, L.B. and DeBusk, R.F. (1983) Effects of early postmyocardial infarction exercise testing on self-perception and subsequent physical activity. *American Journal of Cardiology* 51: 1076–1080.

Finckenor, M. and Byrd-Bredbenner, C. (2000) Nutrition intervention group program based on preaction-stage-oriented change processes of the Transtheoretical Model promotes long-term reduction in dietary fat intake. *Journal of the American Dietetic Association,* 100(3): 335–342.

Fullard, E.M. (1990) Organisation of secondary prevention of coronary heart disease in primary care: the nurse's perspective. *Coronary Health Care* 2: 193–201.

Gambling, T. (2003) A qualitative study into the informational needs of coronary heart disease patients. *International Journal of Health Promotion & Education* 41(3): 68–76.

Grundy, S.M., Balady, G.J., Criqui, M.H., Fletcher, G., Greenland, P., Hiratzka, L.F., Houston-Miller, N., Kris-Etherton, P., Krumhloz, H.M., LaRosa, J., Ockene, I.S., Pearson, T.A., Reed, J., Washington, R. and Smith, S. (1998) Primary Prevention of Coronary Heart Disease: Guidance from Framingham. A statement for healthcare professionals from the AHA Task Force in Risk Reduction. *Circulation* 97: 1876–1887.

Hall Sims, K. and Zucker, D.M. (1999) Smoking cessation. In: Jairath, N. (1999) (ed) *Coronary Heart Disease & Risk Factor Management: A Nursing Perspective.* London: W.B. Saunders.

Hein, E.C. (1998) *Contemporary Leadership Behaviour Selected Readings,* 5th edn. New York: J.B. Lippincott.

Hilton, S., Doherty, S., Kendrick, T., Kerry, S., Rink, E. and Steptoe, A. (1999) Promotion of healthy behaviour among adults at an increased risk of coronary heart disease in general practice: methodology and baseline data from the Change of Heart study. *Health Education Journal* 58: 3–16.

Horgan, J., Bethell, H., Carson, P., Davidson, C., Julian, D., Mayai, R.A. and Nagle, R. (1992) Working party report on cardiac rehabilitation. *British Heart Journal* 61: 412–418.

Houston Miller, N. and Taylor, C.B. (1995) *Lifestyle Management for Patients with Coronary Heart Disease. Current Issues in Cardiac Rehabilitation,* (Series 2). Champaign, IL: Human Kinetics.

Jordan, J.P. and Nigg, C.R. (2002) Applying the transtheoretical model: tailoring interventions to stages of change. In: Burbank, P.M. and Riebe, D. (eds) *Promoting Exercise and Behavior Change in Older Adults Interventions with the Transtheoretical Model.* New York: Springer Publishing Company.

Jue, N.H. and Cunningham, S.L. (1998) Stages of exercise behavior change at two time periods following coronary artery bypass graft surgery. *Cardiovascular Nursing* 13(1): 23–33.

Kristeller, J.L. (1999) Managing smoking as a risk factor in cardiac disease: and educational, behavioral and pharmacologic perspective. In: Rippe, J.M. (ed) *Lifestyle Medicine.* Oxford: Blackwell Science.

Lancaster, T. and Stead, L.F. (2001) Self-help interventions for smoking cessation. *Cochrane Library.* Issue 1, Oxford, Update Software.

Loughlan, C. and Mutrie, N. (1997) An evaluation of the effectiveness of three interventions in promoting physical activity in a sedentary population. *Health Education Journal* 56: 154–165.

Mullen, P.D., Maims, D.A. and Velez, R.V. (1992) A meta analysis of controlled trials of cardiac patient education. *Patient Education and Counseling* 19: 143–162.

Nigg, C.R. and Riebe, D. (2002) The transtheoretical model: research review of exercise behaviour in older adults. In: Burbank, P.M. and Riebe, D. (eds) *Promoting Exercise and*

Behavior Change in Older Adults Interventions with the Transtheoretical Model. New York: Springer Publishing Company.

Orem, D.E. (2001) *Nursing: Concepts of Practice*, 6th edn. London: Mosby.

Priest, V. and Speller, V. (1991) *The Risk Factor Management Manual.* Oxford: Radcliffe Medical Press.

Prochaska, J.O. and DiClemente, C.C. (1982) Transtheoretical therapy: towards a more integrative model of change. *Psychotherapy: Theory, Research and Practice* 19: 276–288.

Prochaska, J.O. and DiClemente, C.C. (1983) Stages and processes of the self-change of smoking: toward an integrative model of change. *Journal of Consulting and Clinical Psychology,* 51(3):390–395.

Prochaska, J.O. and DiClemente, C.C. (1984) *Transtheoretical Approach. Crossing Boundaries of Therapy.* Homewood, IL: Dow-Jones-Irwin.

Prochaska, J.O., DiClemente, C.C. and Norcross, J.C. (1992) In search of how people change applications to addictive behaviours. *American Psychologist* 47(9): 1102–1114.

Prochaska, J.O., Norcross, J.C. and DiClemente, C.C. (1994) *Changing for Good. The Revoluntionary Program That Explains the Six Stages of Change and Teaches You How to Free Yourself from Bad Habits.* New York: William Morrow and Company, Inc.

Pyorälä, K., De Backer, G., Graham, I., Poole Wilson, P. and Wood, D. (1994) Prevention of coronary disease in clinical practice. Recommendations of the task force of the European Society of Cardiology, European Atherosclerosis Society and European Society of Hypertension. *European Heart Journal* 15: 1300–1331.

Quinn, T., Webster, R. and Hatchett, R. (2002) Coronary heart disease: angina and acute myocardial infarction. In: Hatchett, R. and Thompson, D. (eds) *Cardiac Nursing.* London: Harcourt Publishing Ltd.

Rippe, J.M. and O'Brien, D. (1999) The rationale for intervention to reduce the risk of coronary artery disease. In: Rippe, J.M. (ed) *Lifestyle Medicine.* Oxford: Blackwell Science.

Robinson, J. (1991) Project 2000: The role of resistance in the process of professional growth. *Journal of Advanced Nursing*, 16, 820–824.

Rossi, S.R. and Rossi, J.S. (1999) Concepts and theoretical models. In: Jairath, N. (ed) *Coronary Heart Disease & Risk Factor Management: A Nursing Perspective.* London: W.B. Saunders.

Thompson, P. (1999) A review of behaviour change theories in patient compliance to exercise-based rehabilitation following acute myocardial infarction. *Coronary Health Care* 3: 18–24.

Wiles, R. (1994) *Lifestyles Advice in Primary Care.* Southampton: University of Southampton Institute for Health Policy Studies.

Williams, D. (1999) Nursing assessment. In: Jairath, N. (ed) *Coronary Heart Disease & Risk Factor Management: A Nursing Perspective.* London: W.B. Saunders.

Wood, D. (1998) European and American recommendations for coronary heart disease prevention. *European Heart Journal* 19(Suppl A): A12–19.

World Health Organization (2003) *International Cardiovascular Disease Statistics.* (Online). Available at www.who.int/ncd/cvd (accessed 21 November 2003).

Chapter 5

Patient education in coronary care

Key points
• Adult learners need to be actively involved in the education process. • Readiness to learn and previous experience are important considerations when teaching adults. • Assessment of individual patient learning needs is crucial to educational success. • Patient and nurse perception of priority cardiac learning needs differs. • Individualised systematic education programmes are more likely to be effective.

Introduction

Patient education forms an integral component of the role of the nurse in the coronary care unit (CCU). Patients entering the CCU have cardiac disorders that are often life-threatening and this means that they are well disposed to receive education that may improve their chances of living a long and healthy life. Admission to the unit is in itself stressful and patients require orientation and an explanation of what is happening. The provision of education to cardiac patients is thought to reduce stress, aid understanding of their condition and to improve compliance with treatment.

For many patients with coronary heart disease, education regarding lifestyle management can greatly improve their quality of life. In hospitals offering cardiac rehabilitation programmes, education forms part of this process, along with exercise, dietary advice and sometimes counselling. The rehabilitation process is usually structured, following a standardised format consisting of individual or group sessions over a number of weeks and is run by a health professional such as a nurse, doctor or physiotherapist. Patients commence the programme following discharge and a multi-disciplinary approach is commonly preferred.

Cardiac rehabilitation is hugely successful in helping patients to return to normal life and may also prevent the disease from progressing. Although evidence is mounting that cardiac rehabilitation should be widely available to patients, all hospitals do not offer this service, and where the service is offered, not all patients who would benefit from the programme are able to attend. In addition, there are patients who present to the CCU suffering from conditions other than coronary heart disease who may therefore not be invited to attend the rehabilitation sessions. In these situations, the nurse must provide the required education component of the programme at ward level.

Even where structured programmes are available it may be useful for the nurse to provide education to the patient, rather than classifying education as 'someone else's responsibility'. Many benefits can be gained from the provision of education by the nurse in coronary care. First, while rehabilitation programmes have traditionally commenced some weeks after discharge, there is evidence that patients require information before this time. Secondly, the nurse is in a position to provide education to all patients, not just those who may be selected for/or choose to attend rehabilitation. Finally, the nurse is in a prime position to provide individual teaching rather than teaching in groups. This last point is particularly important as information given on the basis of individual need is more likely to be absorbed. Education provided in CCU should not be an isolated event, but rather one stage in a planned, systematic, collegial and seamless approach to equipping patients with the necessary knowledge and skills to promote optimum recovery and realise their full potential.

Education provided in CCU may be recorded in the patient's case notes and built upon during cardiac rehabilitation. It may be useful to use computerised records that may be easily accessed by the rehabilitation services. Patient-held records are also becoming increasingly popular. These may be retained by the patient and taken along to rehabilitation sessions. Increasingly, hospital practice aims towards seamless care and it is important in this regard to transfer education information between the CCU and rehabilitation services. In addition, duplication of education may not be a good use of resources. Communication, through adequate use and transfer of records would reduce the possibility of this.

This chapter examines the concept of patient education in detail. Knowles' (1989) theory of andragogy is described and presented as a suggested framework to build education practices upon.

What is patient education?

There is no universally accepted definition of patient education. It has been described as 'the imparting of information, skills or knowledge with the aim of bringing about changes in patient behavior or attitude' (Luker and Caress 1989) and 'a process which empowers individuals to change behavior, accept health-related information, become partners in their medical regimes and fit new health behaviors into their daily lives' (Smith 1989). Above all, it is an active process that involves the nurse in teaching and the patient in learning. Many teaching methods are used including booklets, lectures, web/computer-based learning, videotape recordings and informal discussion.

Some authors have highlighted the need for the development of an accepted universal theory of health education (Nolan and Nolan 1998). This is based on the belief that sound theory is essential to the design of effective, efficient and practical education programmes (Naidoo and Wills 1994).

However, no definitive theory exists; rather, health education draws on a body of knowledge from a variety of sciences (Scaffa 1998). Barriers to the development of a comprehensive theory are identified as the complexity of human behaviour, the complexity of health behaviours, the difficulties of achieving consensus and acceptance, and lack of perception of the need for, and agreement on, a theory among health educators (Scaffa 1998). Scaffa (1998) suggested that the lack of a clearly defined theory to guide health education stems from the level of development and maturity within the health professions. She termed this a 'pre-paradigm' phase, where instead of a uniform theory to inform practice, there is random activity. This natural phase of professional development and evolution seems to fit with current activities within cardiac patient education.

As an alternative to the pursuit of a uniform methodological approach, Naidoo and Wills (1994) suggest that attention should be focused on the quality of the educational process. This point has also been endorsed by Mullen et al. (1992) who conducted a meta-analysis of controlled trials of cardiac patient education and concluded that effectiveness of education was not determined by a specific technique, but by the quality of planning of the intervention. Mullen et al. (1992) recommended the use of principles such as reinforcement, feedback, individualisation, facilitation and relevance to patients' needs.

These principles are core concepts of Knowles' (1989) theory of andragogy, an adult learning theory. Several authors have suggested that a standard practice based on this theory would enable nurses to understand the conditions required for learning to take place and to enable a commitment to patient education to become effective in practice (Milazzo 1980, Wingate 1990). Rather than simply principles-led practice, a theory such as Knowles' that incorporates such principles would have additional benefits for practice. This includes the capacity to test and develop theory and the ability to integrate multiple theories that inform the nursing situation.

As James and Dickoff (1982) have suggested, we must be liberal and flexible and pluralistic with regard to the application of science and research. In addition to grand theory, James and Dickoff (1982: 25) suggested using 'tiny theories' such as research findings, and they recommended that 'choosing or adopting *a* theory (or conceptual framework) should be replaced by attempts to discern what repertoire of theories should be available for nursing' (James and Dickoff 1982: 24, emphasis is authors' own). Where Orem's self-care deficit nursing theory (2001) is used, for example, teaching is a nursing action where patient self-care deficit exists. Building a knowledge base to inform patient education/teaching might be informed by several theories in addition to research on the topic. It is informative, for instance, to understand how adults learn.

How adults learn

Merriam (1987) stated that if we understand how adults learn we will be able to predict when and how best learning will take place. Several authors concerned with cardiac patient education have suggested that Knowles' theory facilitates this understanding (Milazzo 1980, Gerard and Peterson 1984, Chan 1990, Wingate 1990, Mirka 1994) and andragogy has been used as a framework for patient teaching for a number of years. The andragogical approach suggests that learners are self-directed and draw on their own personal experience (Howard 1993). We should therefore as teachers base learning on the individual's 'need to know' (Jarvis 1985). At the same time, Knowles (1989) has identified four key components of adult learning: self-concept, past experience, readiness to learn, and the diagnosis of learning needs.

Self-concept refers to adult learners having a concept of being responsible for their own decisions (Knowles 1989). In accordance with this principle, information for cardiac patients should be presented in such a way that the patient is directly involved in planning, learning and goal setting (Mirka 1994). The more the adult learner is involved in the planning of their own learning, the more likely it is that their goals will be attained (Mirka 1994). Mutual goal setting fosters self-directed learning skills that are more useful to the patient than information presented in the traditional manner (Knowles 1989).

Past experience has a significant impact on adult learning (Gessner 1989). It can influence patients' perception of events and utilisation of specific coping resources (Mirka 1994). Assessment of the cardiac patient's previous experience of the illness situation and subsequent perception of the healthcare system is crucial (Gessner 1989, Mirka 1994) in assisting the nurse to identify learning needs (Mirka 1994). Knowles (1989) suggests that ignoring the impact of previous experiences on the patient may be a significant barrier to identifying these needs. The patient's previous experience of reading is also crucial. Illiteracy is an identified barrier to learning, and with many teaching materials available only in written format, it can cause serious problems for the patient (Doak et al. 1985). Even where there is no illiteracy as such, many educational reading materials are written in language that is partially incomprehensible to the average patient (Zion and Aiman 1989). The material may also be unsuitable for patients from ethnic minorities, which form large parts of the population in various regions of the UK and indeed of cardiac patient populations (Webster et al. 2002). An accurate assessment of the patient's reading ability is required to ensure that these learning tools are useful. However, this is not always possible, as patients may not admit to a reading deficit. It is important therefore that nursing staff back up written information with verbal information and involve members of the family in teaching sessions. It is also essential that nurses are involved not only in the evaluation of current reading materials in their practice but also in the development of the material, with particular emphasis on ease of understanding and local languages.

Teaching methods may also prove ineffective if the patient is not *ready to learn* (Knowles 1989). Several factors may influence readiness. The motivation of adult learners is generated from internal rather than external sources (Knowles 1989). This intrinsic motivation affects the patient's readiness to learn (Ruzicki 1989). Therefore, how ready a patient is to retain information relies heavily on the patient's internal motivation, rather than specific behaviours of the nurse. This motivation can be affected by the situation the patient is facing. Major life events, such as illness, often act as motivating factors in patient learning (Gessner 1989, Knowles 1989). However, regardless of the life event, individuals may vary in their readiness. Stages of change identified by Prochaska and DiClemente (1982, 1984) as discussed in Chapter 4, may affect this readiness to learn.

The patient in the coronary care unit also presents with many environmental factors that can hinder *readiness to learn*. These include duration and type of illness, treatment modalities and prognosis (Oberst 1989). Physical factors such as pain, fatigue, disability and physiological changes may also seriously impair the patient's ability to retain information (Shea et al. 1985, Ruzicki 1989). Readiness to learn may also be influenced by stage of illness or recovery. Several authors who examined the educational needs of cardiac patients found that the reported needs varied with time (Casey et al. 1984, Gerard and Peterson 1984, Moynihan 1984, Karlik and Yarcheski 1987, Chan 1990, Wingate 1990, Turton 1998, Timmins and Kaliszer 2003). Assessment of the patient's readiness to learn is clearly crucial to the learning process. However, it has received little attention in the application of cardiac patient education programmes (Mirka 1994). In addition, Luker and Caress (1989) suggest that nurses are ill prepared to undertake this kind of assessment on a routine basis, with appropriate training often not provided in basic undergraduate programmes (Luker and Caress 1989).

Diagnosis of learning needs is critical to adult education (Knowles 1989). It involves the following components: assessment of needs; formulation of objectives; the design of learning experiences and evaluation. Current teaching programmes are often based on healthcare workers' perceptions of patients' needs rather than the patients' own perceptions. Wingate (1990) suggests formulating priorities for patient teaching based on an assessment of the patient's critical learning needs. These are the teaching areas that patients perceive as being most important for learning. Scott and Thompson (2003) concur with this view suggesting personal interviews to assess patients' individual needs.

Ruzicki (1989) recognised that there are certain constraints, such as time and resources that militate against the education of short-stay patients by nurses in hospital settings and outlined methods of realistically meeting these patients' learning needs. He suggested that not all patients require the same level of instruction or are ready for instruction. Therefore, in order to provide *realistic* teaching, assessment should be performed in two areas: learning needs (including assessment of previous experience) and readiness to learn.

Assessment of learning needs

Assessment of needs is a crucial component of cardiac patient education programmes (Moynihan 1984, Wingate 1990). Educators have long favoured the 'needs' approach as a means of educating adults (Mason-Attwood and Ellis 1971, Ruzicki 1989). Rather than imparting information based on the preferences of administration, or implementing mass programmes designed for general use, this approach attempts to identify and meet the needs of the individual. Knowles (1989) defines a learning need as the gap between competencies specified and the present level of development by the learner. The crucial element in the assessment of the 'gap' is the learner's own perception of the discrepancy between where they are now and where they want to be (Knowles 1989). Suggested methods for assessing needs include observation, listening, communication skills, discussions with family members, use of the patient records and documentation, with an emphasis on the practicality of methods used (Ruzicki 1989). Assessment of the patient's previous hospital/healthcare or illness experience is also an important component of assessment, as these experiences may affect the needs (Ruzicki 1989).

To guide patient teaching in the CCU it is also helpful to have a framework of cardiac patients' generalised learning needs. Exploring research on the topic concurs with James and Dickoff's (1982) notion of merging tiny theories and research to develop a knowledge base for particular practices. Knowledge of what cardiac patients in general need to know following acute cardiac events and subsequent admission to CCU can be useful for developing learning needs assessment tools. Each individual patient can be presented with the generalised needs in the area and may choose which areas he or she requires more knowledge about. This framework may be developed from the literature in the area.

Several studies have addressed the learning needs of cardiac patients (Casey et al. 1984, Gerard and Peterson 1984, Moynihan 1984, Karlik and Yarcheski 1987, Chan 1990, Wingate 1990, Jaarsma et al. 1995, Turton 1998, Timmins and Kaliszer 2003). Many of these examined needs from both the nurse's and the patient's perspective, and one also examined the spouses' view (Turton 1998). There is general agreement in the literature about the learning needs of cardiac patients. Perceived needs exist in the areas of psychological factors, risk (lifestyle) factors, medication information, information on diet and physical activity, cardiac anatomy and physiology and orientation to the CCU environment (Casey et al. 1984, Gerard and Peterson 1984, Moynihan 1984, Karlik and Yarcheski 1987, Chan 1990, Wingate 1990, Jaarsma et al. 1995, Turton 1998). Management of symptoms also emerged as priority learning in recent studies (Turton 1998, Timmins and Kaliszer 2003).

There is little evidence outlining the extent to which this specific information is provided to patients in the CCU and it is most likely that it is still provided as Moynihan (1984) described – on a 'sporadic' basis. Indeed Jaarsma et al.'s (1995) study suggested that by their own account most patients had a knowledge deficit and required more information in the areas of risk factors, deleterious effects of treatment, convalescence and knowledge of their disease. A recent study of the experiences of Gujarati Hindu patients in the first month following myocardial infarction (MI) revealed 'lack of information' as an emerging theme (Webster et al. 2002). A similar picture emerged in Thompson et al. (1995) and Gambling's (2003) studies. 'It was apparent that when advice and information was given to patients, it was perceived to be vague and inadequate or did not meet the patients' or partners' expectations in some way' (Thompson et al. 1995).

While there is general agreement about what 'should be taught' to patients, it is clear that in practice careful consideration is required of patients' individual needs and readiness to learn in these areas. Individual patient needs vary over time. Priority learning areas post discharge have been found to be quite different from those expressed during the hospital stay. The only exception to this was risk (lifestyle) factors that remained as priority learning except in one study (Moynihan 1984) where patients did not view this as important while in the CCU. Needs also differed for patients who had myocardial infarction for the first time; these patients placed greater emphasis on learning of risk factors (Casey et al. 1984).

The most important finding in many of these studies is that while there is general agreement between patients and nurses regarding general learning needs, they have significantly different views on what constitutes priority learning. Many patients perceived the area of risk (lifestyle) factors to be of greatest importance (Gerard and Peterson 1984, Karlik and Yarcheski 1987, Chan 1990, Wingate 1990, Turton 1998) whereas nursing staff often deemed this to be of lesser importance (Gerard and Peterson 1984, Karlik and Yarcheski 1987). Some nurses perceived medication information to be of greatest importance to patients (Casey et al. 1984, Gerard and

Peterson 1984) in contrast with patients who placed a low priority on this area, particularly in the early stages of recovery (Wingate 1990). Under the category 'activity' nurses perceived 'resuming sexual activity' to be of high importance, whereas patients viewed this as being of low importance (Turton 1998, Timmins and Kaliszer 2003).

These findings indicate that patients appear to favour practical information about their condition, its cause and prevention, whereas nurses are more focused on medical aspects of care such as medications and anatomy and physiology, although one recent study has indicated more agreement between nurse and patient views than previously reported (Timmins and Kaliszer 2003). Symptom management was a top priority for both groups. However, for individual items significant differences still emerged, particularly with regard to activity. The discrepancies noted in all the studies may be due to the fact that during illness patients view information central to their survival as being of the highest importance and perhaps does not fully understand the importance of teaching in certain areas such as medications and activity. Patients appeared to be very focused on symptom management so it is essential that patients' needs be assessed in this area in particular and specific teaching interventions provided.

Medication advice, although it does not come out strongly as a patient priority, must be recognised as a *nursing need*. Patients clearly need advice and explanation in this area; in Jaarsma et al.'s (1995) study more than half of the patients discharged suffered effects of treatment post discharge and 23% of patients required further information in the area of medications. What may be required during assessment of needs in this area is negotiation with the patient to ensure that the nurse's (i.e. teacher's) need to provide crucial information is retained. It is important to remember to avoid routine information giving in this area. Although medications are a nursing priority, individual patient assessment may reveal that some patients actually require little information as a result of prior knowledge, whereas others may require a lot of support to achieve knowledge and understanding. Written materials are important to support this teaching.

It is of interest that receiving information on medication was rated highly in one recent study (Timmins and Kaliszer 2003), perhaps indicating an increased public awareness about medication and less passivity towards their use. Scott and Thompson (2003) commented on the possible increase in public awareness with today's patients regarded as 'more active, assertive consumers of healthcare'.

Resuming sexual activity is another area where the nurse's and patient's priorities differ. Cardiac nurses often provide advice to patients about this area on a routine basis. As studies have indicated, this area is often of low priority to patients, particularly in the early stages of recovery, it is essential that patients' individual needs be used to guide the teaching process. Again, nurses may need to provide patients with basic information quite briefly following negotiation, leaving plenty of time for other areas which patients view as more important. The difficulty is that although issues relating to the resumption of sexual activity have been identified as an area to which cardiac nurses should give *more* priority to (Whitaker 2000), it is clearly not the view of some patients in their care. The important factor in teaching in this area is individual needs assessment; for many patients this may be a critical factor in their recovery, whereas others may have little or no need for information on this topic due to their own personal circumstances. As an alternative to sexual activity as a topic, sexuality as an area could be explored during assessment of self-care requisites. This topic has been little examined in the published literature and further research is required to illuminate patients' needs in this area.

Ruzicki (1989) was quite critical of the teaching that cardiac nurses provided, stating that patients are often given highly technical information while in hospital that is often of little use to them. Nurses traditionally teach physiologically-based topics to patients. However, Ruzicki (1989) states that during the short hospital stay only important 'survival information' should be taught. This is supported by the effect of the addition of one section 'symptom management' to the Cardiac Patients Learning Needs Inventory (CPLNI) (Gerard and Peterson, 1984) by Turton (1998). This tool, used to collect data in many studies of patient learning needs, was adapted during the validation process, which included a pilot study. The additional section, which contained items such as 'What to do if I get chest pain', 'The signs and symptoms of a heart attack' and 'When to call a GP or ambulance', emerged as priority learning for patients, spouses and nurses in both Turton's (1998) and Timmins' and Kaliszer's (2003) study.

A limitation of the information in this area is that the identified needs are mainly a reflection of patient groups such as those who have undergone CABG, MI or angioplasty. Little information is available for other patient groups who may present to CCU. Patients with coronary heart disease, who have not proceeded to MI may have similar needs to those described.

In summary teaching in the CCU should therefore consider patients' needs for priority information and avoid undue focus on aspects of care that are of little importance to patients. Individual needs assessment should focus on the main areas identified in the literature: CCU environment, anatomy and physiology, psychological factors/emotional reactions, risk (lifestyle) factors, general activity and medications. A teaching plan and individual goals can then be devised based on the individual preferences in each area, and on nurse/patient negotiation. Time may be provided during the assessment to allow the patient to state individual needs that have not already been taken into account. This complies with the suggestions of a recent systematic review of needs assessment of patients with MI (Scott and Thompson 2003).

A sample assessment framework is provided in Figure 5.1. As well as providing information for tailored individual education programmes, the use of written assessment tools such as this allows for accurate documentation, an important consideration in today's healthcare environment. This assessment framework may be used during an informal interview to compile the joint needs of the patient and their spouse or partner. A simply designed assessment form is necessary for speed and ease of completion. Needs assessment tools are common in the research literature but are cumbersome for regular in-patient needs assessment. Many of these tools use Likert scales, requiring the patient to rate the importance of the item on a scale ranging from 'not important' to 'very important'. These ratings of importance are not required in CCU assessment in which all items are of importance. They have also been found not to be very discriminating (Timmins and Kaliszer 2003, Scott and Thompson 2003). Simple yes/no statements are sufficient, allowing easy analysis.

Patient name:			Date of admission:
Spouse/partner name:			Date of assessment:
Patient hospital number:			
Previous experience with this illness:			Comments:
Previous hospital admission with cardiac event	Y/N		
Previous hospital admission/experience	Y/N		
Previous history of cardiac disorder	Y/N		
Relevant knowledge related to this disorder	Y/N		

Other relevant previous experience:			Comments:
Good knowledge of the English language	Y/N		
Good reading knowledge of the English language	Y/N		
Usefulness of reading materials	Y/N		
Learning needs in specific areas: patient (P) spouse/partner/family (S)			

Information required about risk factors/lifestyle:	P	S	Comments
Contribution of risk factors to the development of CHD	Y/N	Y/N	
Smoking	Y/N	Y/N	
Diet/obesity	Y/N	Y/N	
Raised serum cholesterol	Y/N	Y/N	
Diabetes	Y/N	Y/N	
Hypertension	Y/N	Y/N	
Other:	Y/N	Y/N	

Information required about orientation to the CCU:			Comments
General environment	Y/N	Y/N	
Beside equipment	Y/N	Y/N	
Unit equipment	Y/N	Y/N	
Visiting times	Y/N	Y/N	
Usual routine	Y/N	Y/N	
Visitor facilities	Y/N	Y/N	
Family support	Y/N	Y/N	

Information required about the cardiac disorder and related anatomy and physiology:			Comments:
Structure and function of the normal heart and coronary circulation	Y/N	Y/N	
Structure and function of normal cardiac conduction system	Y/N	Y/N	
Structure and function of the circulatory system	Y/N	Y/N	
Physiology related to personal condition	Y/N	Y/N	
Manifestations and symptoms of current condition	Y/N	Y/N	
Treatment modalities related to current condition	Y/N	Y/N	

Information required about emotional reactions:			Comments:
Common reactions to illness	Y/N	Y/N	
Expression of fears and feelings	Y/N	Y/N	
Ways of coping with stress	Y/N	Y/N	
Adjusting to life with cardiac disease	Y/N	Y/N	

Information required about medication:			Comments:
General advice and explanation about medication	Y/N	Y/N	
General rules about medication, including timing	Y/N	Y/N	
Adverse effects of medication	Y/N	Y/N	
Steps to be taken if side effects to medication occur	Y/N	Y/N	
Becoming familiar with new medication	Y/N	Y/N	
The importance of compliance	Y/N	Y/N	

Information required about physical activity:			Comments:
Balance between activity and rest	Y/N	Y/N	
Advice about work/housekeeping	Y/N	Y/N	
Advice about social activities	Y/N	Y/N	
Advice about driving	Y/N	Y/N	
Advice about sexual activity	Y/N	Y/N	

Information required about symptom management:			Comments:
Explanation of main symptoms of the disorder	Y/N	Y/N	
Explanation about the signs and symptoms of a heart attack	Y/N	Y/N	
Consequences of condition on daily life	Y/N	Y/N	
Control of symptoms	Y/N	Y/N	
When to call a GP or ambulance	Y/N	Y/N	
Patient support groups	Y/N	Y/N	

| **Other patient/family perceived learning needs:** | | | Comments: |

Figure 5.1 Cardiac patients learning needs assessment: a sample assessment framework.

Emotional needs

Risk factor education may be offered to many patients as a component of primary prevention and emotional reactions are likely to be present with many conditions. Psychological factors/emotional support for cardiac patients requires particular attention. The hospital admission may be a daunting prospect for many, especially those for whom it is the first time. In addition, there may be extra stress associated with having a condition related to the heart, which has clear associations with life and death for the patient. These factors may result in patient anxiety and depression, and generalised emotional turmoil. Although this has been recognised by some professionals in the field, such as Thompson (1989) and Jowett and Thompson (2000), who recommend in-hospital counselling for coronary patients, the support that patients receive in this area is far from ideal. Where cardiac rehabilitation programmes exist, patients may receive support from a counsellor or psychologist, although programmes do not always follow standardised guidelines and the nature of support personnel varies between programmes. In addition, some hospitals do not operate these programmes and many patients either do not attend or are not suitable for attendance, due to the nature of their condition. The first step in providing education and support for patients in this area is to establish patients' learning needs in general, which can then be adapted for specific situations.

Studies indicate that patients experience significant emotional adjustment during the recovery period following acute cardiac events; feelings of *loss of control* for the patient may result in anxiety and depression. However, patients' learning needs in this area have not been clearly identified (Jaarsma et al. 1995). Studies that have examined cardiac patients' learning needs have found that most patients perceive 'psychological factors' or 'emotional response' to be of importance to learn, particularly in the early stages of recovery (Gerard and Peterson 1984, Moynihan 1984, Chan 1990, Wingate 1990, Turton 1998, Timmins and Kaliszer 2003). However, when placed in rank order with other learning needs, patients rated this area below risk factors, medication, physical activity and anatomy and physiology. The only exception to these findings is in the research of Karlik and Yarcheski (1987) who found that patients considered this area to be of low importance both in hospital and while at home, and rated it last compared with other learning needs.

Jaarsma *et al.* (1995) outlined the problems experienced by 82 cardiac patients 6 months after discharge. Their findings revealed that 59% of patients experienced emotional reactions. The presence of these problems differed significantly between the three groups of patients (those who had undergone CABG (n=23), those who had MI (n=24), and those who had CABG and a previous history of MI (n=35). A significant finding was that 79% of MI patients experienced reactions when compared with the other two patient groups. Survivors of a first time MI appeared to experience greater emotional impact than their peers who were undergoing major surgical procedures.

However, beyond these generalisations of emotional needs, and referral to specific mood states such as anxiety and depression, there is little description of the emotional reactions of patients following acute events and their needs in this area. Anxiety and depression are reported as common experiences in patients who have had acute coronary events such as MI (Stern et al. 1977, Wiklund et al. 1984, Lewin et al. 1992, Ladwig et al. 1994). The experience of these two states may actually impede patient recovery and their ability to return to their previous independence. Conn et al. (1991) revealed that depression accounted for 49% of the variance in quality of life among 94 older patients who had had an MI. Depression scores also predicted behavior in areas such as risk factor reduction. Depression has also been associated with a greater mortality and morbidity from coronary heart disease (Dobbels *et al.* 2002). Depression and anxiety have an obvious impact on the recovery of patients with MI, although its impact on other patient groups is less well understood. Early diagnosis and treatment are therefore a crucial adjunct to usual care for these patient groups. It is imperative that the nurse alerts the medical personnel to any signs of irritability, fatigue, malaise, anger and anxiety in patients in their care. Early medical intervention allows prompt diagnosis of the conditions and early pharmacological and psychological interventions that may be prescribed on an individual basis for patients (Dobbels *et al.* 2002).

Supportive-educative counselling, as a component of a nurse-led structured in-hospital education programme may also be of benefit to patients suffering from anxiety and depression. Using a quasi-experimental approach, Thompson (1989) demonstrated a significant reduction in anxiety and depression among 60 patients with first time MI following supportive-educative nurse counselling. Lewin et al. (1992) demonstrated similar results with 176 patients.

Supportive-educative counselling may also be of benefit in supporting patients with measurable anxiety and depressive states and as most patients express 'needs' in the psychological/emotional area, it is likely that all patients would benefit from this provision.

Patients appear to experience of 'loss of control' over their lives after an acute cardiac event. Johnston and Morse (1990) examined the process of adjustment that 14 individuals experienced following an MI. Qualitative analysis revealed the process of adjustment whereby individuals struggled to regain a sense of control over their lives. In the initial hospital phase patients exhibited the first of four phases, 'defending oneself', where they used coping strategies such as denial to keep this sense of control.

This loss can affect later psychological adjustment. Moser and Dracup (1995) described the relationship between 176 patients' feelings of control after an acute cardiac event and psychological recovery at 6 months. Those patients who had a greater sense of control were less anxious, depressed and hostile and were better adjusted psychosocially than those with low control.

Clearly, emotional support for patients needs to incorporate aspects of education to increase the perceived control over events. Emotional needs often do not receive high priority when considering the learning needs of patients within coronary care. In their meta-analysis of 1992 Mullen et al. revealed that of the 28 studies that fulfilled the eligibility criteria, only three programmes had interventions aimed at reducing emotional stress. Areas regarding risk factor reduction received much higher priority as nurses focused on technical aspects of care. Interventions to promote mental health need to become an integral component of formal education programmes (Conn et al. 1991).

The families of patients who have had an acute coronary event also need to be included in mental health interventions. It has been shown that spouses of patients with MI experience a wide range of emotions in response to their partner's illness. Thompson et al. (1995) noticed that partners mounted a type of surveillance activity, watching their partner in an overprotective way. Many spouse/partner fears emerged such as fear of further events. The two in a factor analysis by Kettuen et al. (1999) were disease-related fears and personal fears. Interestingly, these fears were not directly related to the severity of the event, but rather the occurrence of the event. In this study spouse support lessened the existence of fears. Turton (1998) revealed that information needs of cardiac patients and their spouses were broadly similar, although they differed from those of the nursing staff. Kettuen et al. (1999) suggested that assessment of individual needs and provision of support be extended to family members, and that education programmes be tailored to individual *families* rather than being driven by the health service entirely.

Learning needs and conceptual models

Use of nursing theory and conceptual models of nursing as suggested in the first three chapters of this book is also useful to develop supportive-educative systems for cardiac patients. The conceptual model (Orem 2001) that features in Chapters 2 and 3 highlights the important role that nurses have in supporting and educating patients and families. Indeed, Jaarsma (1999) developed a supportive-educative model for heart failure patients on the basis of Orem's model. Integrating this conceptual model into coronary care nursing raises awareness about the fundamental role that nurses have in relation to supporting and educating cardiac patients. It also creates an awareness of the individuality of patients' needs and suggests a new paradigm in educational terms, 'self-care deficit' which has philosophical parity with the needs-driven approach advocated by contemporary educational theorists.

Developing conceptual models for use at local level can involve the integration of relevant and useful theory, consistent with what James and Dickoff (1982) termed theoretical pluralism. As a discipline struggling for credibility in an academic environment, there is a tendency to embrace notions for nursing almost singularly. As an alternative, we need to investigate, develop and harness the research and theory that are required to inform our practice. As James and Dickoff (1982) suggested, we must be liberal and flexible and pluralistic with regard to the application of science and research.

This approach may be conceptualised as a *matrix* that may guide practice (James and Dickoff 1982). James and Dickoff (1982) suggested that grand theory supplies the vertical items on the matrix and typologies of various origins supply the horizontal. Using a matrix approach serves to identify those items that are 'only emerging in the consciousness of the practitioner, theorist or other enquirer' (James and Dickoff 1982: 26). Cardiac nurses should be prepared to integrate several relevant theoretical frameworks to develop quality educational programmes.

Readiness to learn

Readiness to learn has been identified as an important component of adult learning (Knowles 1989). Ruzicki (1989) suggests that assessment of the hospitalised patients' readiness to learn is a crucial component of the in-patient educational process. She suggests that 'not all patients are ready to learn' (Ruzicki 1989) and questions whether valuable nursing time should be spent providing information to patients who are not ready. For those who are not ready and those who are unwilling it is suggested that needs assessment and level of readiness is documented and the patient referred to appropriate services if the reluctance to participate is potentially life threatening.

Readiness to learn can be assessed under the headings of factors affecting educational readiness as identified by Ruzicki (1989). These are physical, socioeconomic, intellectual and psychological. Physical factors include condition, pain, fatigue, disability and sensory deprivation. Socioeconomic factors include financial concerns, home environment, relationships and social support. Intellectual factors include literacy and ability to comprehend and psychological factors include emotional response to illness and beliefs about health. The majority of these factors can easily be assessed using information from the patient, their family and the patient record. However, psychological factors that affect a patient's readiness to learn can be more complex. It is important also for the nurse to understand individual differences in health behaviour and a number of theoretical models have been constructed to explain this phenomenon (Russell 1999).

The most widely referred to is the health belief model; it was initially developed by Hochbaum in the USA while working on the detection and prevention of tuberculosis (Rosenstock 1974a). The model was further developed (Rosenstock 1974b) and later modified by co-researchers Janz and Becker (1984). Hijeck (1984) suggested that the health belief model has direct application to the nursing care of cardiac patients. Hijeck (1984) acknowledged the great amount of time that nurses dedicate to the teaching of cardiac patients and suggested that many nurses remembered those who were unwilling or unable to modify their behaviours. Hijeck suggested that nurses should investigate the factors that influence that decision.

The four categories of the health belief model – perceived susceptibility to disease, perceived benefits of and barriers to preventative care, and cues to action – incorporate the patient's health attitudes, beliefs, current situation and psychological variables (Hijeck 1984). For example, the likelihood of taking preventative action is increased when an individual has a sense of *perceived susceptibility* to disease. This category relates to the extent to which the patient believes that he or she can contract the disease. Hijeck (1984) applied this model to patients with MI, and noticed that their beliefs about the possibility of having a second MI directly related to their perceived susceptibility. *Perceived severity* relates to the extent to which a person believes that their condition is a serious one and this also affects their health behaviour.

The model also predicts that the likelihood of engaging in health protective behaviour is influenced by the perceived *costs versus benefits* of taking a particular course of action. The monetary cost of care and cost of time and inconvenience and the effect the action has on lifestyle may affect the level of engagement. The model also suggests that certain stimuli may function as *cues to action*, increasing the likelihood of engaging in protective behavior, whilst others may function as *barriers to action*, decreasing the likelihood. Hijeck (1984) suggested that the more benefits the patient perceives from the care, the more likely it is that the patient will take action; conversely the more barriers they perceive, the less likely they will take action.

Hijeck (1984) suggests that the cardiac nurse should investigate each of the four categories, identifying the beliefs in each and determine which beliefs will support or inhibit lifestyle modification. The coronary care nurse could use the health belief model to determine early in the hospital stay the probability of the patient's participation and desire to alter lifestyle. Hijeck (1984) also suggested that ascertaining the patient's beliefs might provide the nurse in the CCU with information that could guide planning of educational care. This is aimed at strengthening the patient's decision to attend formal education or adhere to lifestyle changes.

Documentation of the patient's readiness to learn is an important aspect of their care. Figure 5.2 outlines a sample assessment framework that may be used to assess patient readiness. It allows for the assessment of the physiological, psychological, socio-economic and intellectual factors that may reduce a patient's readiness to learn. It also incorporates assessment of the patient's health beliefs. All of these areas can provide vital information to the nurse who can then plan educational interventions based on the patient's state of readiness.

Patient name: Date of admission:
Spouse/partner name: Date of assessment:
Patient hospital number:
Assessment of readiness to learn: Comments:
Physiological/psychological condition
Is the patient's condition stable?   Y/N
Is the patient receiving narcotic analgesia?   Y/N
Is the patient suffering from an underlying psychiatric disorder? Y/N
Is the patient conscious?   Y/N
Is the patient suffering pain?   Y/N

Socio-economic factors/intellectual capacity: Comments:
Does the patient report any socio-economic factors that negate against
receiving cardiac teaching?   Y/N
Does the patient suffer from intellectual disability that may impede teaching? Y/N
Does the patient have sufficient intellectual capacity to receive cardiac
teaching in its current format?   Y/N

Beliefs about health: Comments:
Does the patient perceive their condition to be serious?   Y/N
Does the patient perceive any benefits associated with adaptation to a new
lifestyle?   Y/N
Does the patient perceive that the costs of adaptation to a new lifestyle
outweigh the costs?   Y/N
Can the patient identify barriers to their actions in managing their own health?
(Describe)   Y/N
Can the patient identify 'cues to action' that may exist that may encourage the
patient towards taking the required action? (Describe)   Y/N

Stages of change: Comments:
Pre-contemplation   Y/N
Contemplation   Y/N
Preparation   Y/N
Action   Y/N
Maintenance   Y/N

Figure 5.2 Framework for assessing cardiac patients' readiness to learn.

Role of the nurse in patient education in coronary care

Patient education is increasingly being recognised as an important function in nursing practice (Noble 1991). It forms an integral component of healthcare. It is a process of assisting individuals to change behaviour. Nurses provide patients with information about health, and are encouraged to become partners in their care. As nurses spend a considerable amount of time in direct patient care, several opportunities for patient education arise. This is particularly true of the CCU, where there is often an increased staff/patient ratio compared with hospital wards. As discussed above orientation to the CCU, information about condition, risk factors (lifestyle factors), medications, cardiac anatomy and physiology are areas where information is commonly provided to patients. Emotional factors may also be considered, although these are less commonly included.

Nursing staff utilise a variety of teaching aids to provide this information, including videos and booklets and providing individual teaching to patients. Approaches to teaching can vary. So too can level and content. In the past cardiac in-patient education was often regarded as unplanned and haphazard with effectiveness uncertain (Close 1988); cardiac teaching programmes were often unstructured. In addition, lack of a systematic and individualised approach to teaching, failure to identify a patient's individual learning needs, inappropriate timing of information delivery and inappropriate teaching strategies further contributed to lack of success.

To overcome these barriers, adult learning theory such as Knowles' andragogy (1989) needs to underpin the educational approaches to patient teaching within the CCU. Knowles views the learner as unique, self-motivated and capable of diagnosing his or her own learning needs. This is in complete contrast to many current approaches to patient education that are often nurse-led, routine and standardised. However, literature on this topic indicates that individualising programmes is a key to success. This does not mean that the programmes employed have to be haphazard, on the contrary a standard teaching package can be devised containing the core elements of cardiac education and this can be adapted to suit each patient. Ideally information technology needs to be used, so that the unique teaching programme can be readily prepared. The key to the provision of adequate in-patient teaching is the use of structure to support the teaching process.

Structure provides the framework for patient teaching, thus making it easier for nurses to teach (Ruzicki 1989). Structure may be established through the use of learning theory to support education and the development of standardised patient education programmes, with carefully defined objectives, consistent teaching methods and clear documentation and evaluation methods. The advantages of these programmes are that the nurse has a clearly outlined path of action to follow once learning needs have been established. It also allows for quick documentation, as written/printed plans are readily available. Although standardised patient education programmes are based on generalised needs of large groups of patients, they can be easily adapted to suit individual patients needs. In addition, in an area such as cardiology many learning needs have been established in this group and moreover, many learning areas such as risk factors/lifestyle factors are not only approved by patients but universally recommended by medical authorities and therefore should feature in educational programmes. Standardised programmes need to be realistic and easy to use (Ruzicki 1989). Objectives should focus on need to know (survival) content, so that content can be absorbed during hospital stay. Evaluation of learning can be achieved through verbal assessment, physical observation of a skill or written assessment.

Although not explicitly stated a four-stage model (assess-plan-implement-evaluate) underpins the application of Knowles (1989) theory of andragogy in the practical setting. Table 5.1 outlines the core components of this process. CCU nurses may use this model as a visual representation of the educational process required for cardiac patients.

It is important that the CCU nurse is adequately prepared to undertake their teaching role. This role requires an understanding of theory and its application as well as the communication skills required to complete a successful assessment. Negotiation skills are also required as there may be information that the CCU nurse *needs* to or is required to provide to patients, although the patient may not be aware of the importance or the relevance of this particular area.

The educational process: assessment

The first step in preparing an individual teaching programme for a patient is assessment of the patient's learning needs and readiness to learn. Assessment requires the nurse to be highly skilled at communication as well as knowledgeable in the theory of adult learning (Mirka 1994). The assessment should be a collaborative one, where a nurse–patient relationship develops and patients are encouraged to identify their needs in conjunction with the nurse. Patients' learning needs in the areas commonly taught to cardiac patients (see Figure 5.1) can be identified and documented. Their readiness to learn may also be documented (see Figure 5.2) to include their beliefs about health. Documentation and referral are also important in the teaching process as these enable decisions taken to be easily accessed and understood by other professionals and also allows for accountability.

Planning

Planning the educational process is based on the initial assessment of patient learning needs. Mutually agreed individual goals are set for each patient and standardised teaching packages from chosen areas may be chosen to support the plan. Main teaching areas are identified and arrangements are made to include the family if appropriate. Referral to other sources is essential where patients require additional emotional support, support with bereavement, support with smoking cessation or where the patient does not appear to be ready to learn and failure of self-help could be detrimental to his or her health.

Implementation

Implementation of the education process also involves the use of personal communication, printed materials and web-based learning if appropriate. Mullen et al. (1992) found that the communication channel used had little effect on the outcome of cardiac education. This factor emerges consistently in the literature. There is no *best*

Table 5.1 The educational process in the coronary care unit (CCU)

Assess	Plan	Implement	Evaluate

Self-care requisites
Learning needs
Previous experience
Readiness to learn
Confidence
	Set realistic goals
	Provide standard information
	according to needs on:
	  orientation to CCU
	  risk factors/lifestyle
	  anatomy and physiology/
	    condition
	  medication
	  activity/exercise
	  weight and diet
	Involve family
	Referral to other sources
		Personalised programme
		  tailored to needs
		Provide individualised information
		  and educative counselling support
		  by teaching strategies:
		  structured teaching
		  one to one
		  booklets
		  computer based
		Involve family
			Effectiveness of teaching and learning
			  outcome by assessment of:
			  knowledge level
			  specific behaviours if appropriate
			assess whether or not goals were
			  achieved
			willingness to adapt to lifestyle changes

method of teaching patients. Factors such as individualisation of programmes, reinforcement, relevance and feedback emerge as greater contributors to educational success. In relation to the use of media in particular, relevance is of great importance. Printed materials are often used by nurses when teaching patients and are useful for providing patients and family with reference material, or to reinforce material that has been taught, and are also useful to allow the patient to absorb material in their own time. Ruzicki (1989: 633) comments, however, that these pamphlets are often 'front-loaded with pathophysiology, so that the patient never gets to the important sections'. In addition, they are often directed at adults with a great deal of literacy and comprehension, who do not represent the average patient. Ruzicki (1989) suggests that written material should be checked for simplicity and clarity and should contain 'need to know' information only. It should also be visually attractive with opportunity for patient interaction, to enable them to individualise the content. Non-printed materials, such as audio and video programmes as well as computer-based packages should also be made attractive and relevant to patients. It is vital therefore that the nurse assesses the adequacy and suitability of all media aids used in the implementation process with each patient.

Evaluation

Evaluation is the final stage in the process, which ascertains whether goals have been achieved. It also allows patients to provide feedback about the programme that can be used to alter goals for the patient or to improve the educational process in general.

However, evaluation is a frequently omitted component of the educational process in the practice setting. It is often thought that the provision of education alone is sufficient to provide the patient with the skills and knowledge that are required. Once the teaching has been provided there is a sense that the nurse's responsibility has been met. However, it is essential that evaluation be performed to ensure that the patient has reached a level of knowledge that is sufficient and compares favourably with set goals. Knowles (1989) highlighted evaluation of learning outcomes as a key component in adult learning. Evaluation of the programme may also refer to measuring the success of approaches used and receiving feedback from both patient and family that may improve future programmes. Patient feedback should be encouraged in all stages of the process, to involve the patient and to continuously evaluate a programme's effectiveness.

Evaluation also allows the nurse to pass on information about the success or failure of the process to health professionals who will continue the education once the patient has left the CCU. This may include nursing staff from general/cardiac wards, rehabilitation officers, specialist nurses, community nurses and general practitioners. Evaluation of true educational effectiveness involves a measure of behaviour change as well as an increase in knowledge. In the CCU behaviour in areas such as diet and smoking cannot be fully measured and this needs to be done after discharge. In the CCU the patient is still under hospital restrictions that prevent 'normal' everyday behaviour. However, some behaviour can be evaluated, such as proficiency in medication delivery.

It is important to remember that the acquisition of knowledge does not necessarily result in behaviour change. For example it has been shown that providing information about smoking may not necessarily result in smoking cessation. Explanation about medications does not necessarily result in compliance. It is very clear that providing patients with structured education programmes has the ability to improve their knowledge of the area, but studies where both behaviour and knowledge were examined have highlighted the fact that an increase in knowledge does not necessarily produce changes in behaviour (Barbarowicz et al. 1980, Scalzi et al. 1980, Milazzo 1980, Sivarajan et al. 1983, Fletcher 1987).

Duyree (1992) reviewed the studies on this topic and found that where behavioural change was achieved, this effect was usually limited to one area of behaviour despite education being given on several areas, such as smoking, diet and exercise. Mullen et al. (1992) endorsed this point and concluded that while structured educational programmes have been successful in making an impact on some areas of lifestyle such as exercise and diet, other areas have been affected less consistently. These findings indicate that the relationship between knowledge and behaviour is complex. Achieving long-term success in changing patient behaviour is not a simple process, to be lightly undertaken. Effective education of cardiac patients in the CCU requires a consistent, systematic, collaborative approach. Programmes need careful planning as well as an understanding of patient education, how adults learn, barriers to adopting health behaviours and models for delivery of education.

It is clear that structured educational programmes can achieve success in increasing patients' knowledge and behaviour. Factors identified as effective in eliciting the necessary lifestyle changes include the implementation of teaching programmes that are timely, systematic and individualised (Barbarowicz et al. 1980, Gerard and Peterson 1984, Karlik and Yarcheski 1987, Chan 1990, Horgan et al. 1992, Mirka 1994).

Summary and conclusions

Throughout this chapter, the amalgamation of several theories to inform practical nursing has been discussed. Figure 5.3 is a graphical representation of the philosophical merging of theory and research discussed in this and previous chapters to inform cardiac patient education. Through the understanding of the nursing situation developed in Chapter 2, Orem's (2001) model informs us that the patient has universal, developmental and healthcare deviation needs. Through careful assessment, a self-care deficit with regard to knowledge is identified. Supportive-educative nursing action is required to address this. This framework acknowledges that the patient has beliefs about health, readiness, need to know, self-concept, previous experience (Knowles 1989) that are personal and relevant to the assessment, planning, implementation and evaluation of teaching. The patient can also be classified according to his or her stage of change (Prochaska and DiClemente 1982, 1984; see Chapter 4). Readiness to learn is also influenced by beliefs about health and these need to be considered (Hijeck 1984).

Patient education is a key function of the CCU nurse, as a component of on-going patient care. Many patients entering the CCU require education and advice and the nurse is in a prime position to reciprocate this need. Patient education does not simply mean the imparting of information on a routine basis or the routine

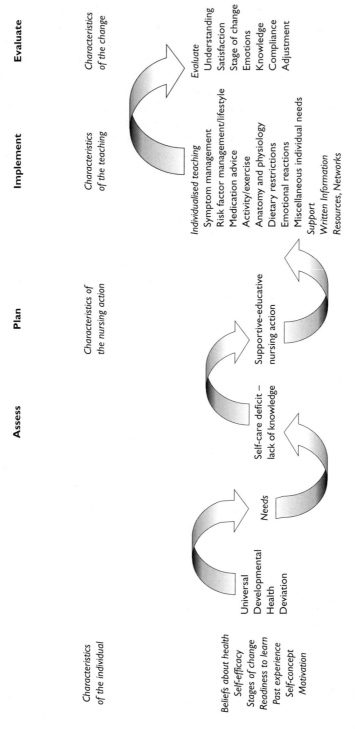

Figure 5.3 A supportive-educative framework to guide cardiac patient education.

distribution of reading materials. Rather, careful consideration must be given to the understanding of how adults learn (Knowles 1989) and barriers that exist to learning, in order to ensure that learning are meaningful and effective. Patients need to be actively involved in the assement of their learning needs and setting of realistic goals. It is no longer appropriate that patients are passive recipients of care in this area.

The needs of patients in the CCU centre primarily on information that is pertinent to survival, including symptom management, psychological factors, risk factor (lifestyle) factors, medication information, information on diet and physical activity, cardiac anatomy and physiology and orientation to the CCU environment. For the most part nurses working in cardiac fields are in agreement with the existence of learning needs in these areas. However, what constitutes priority learning can vary between patients and nurses. This has important implications for the way in which education is delivered, as the nurse may be inclined to teach the patient what they *think* the patient needs to know, rather than what the patient *actually* needs to know. Providing education to patients on an individual basis, tailored to their individual needs is the only way to rectify this situation.

Patient education programmes need to be structured, systematic and well documented. The adoption of needs-based educational programmes in CCU that are timely, systematic and individualised are crucial to achieving the ultimate aim of effective patient education, thereby facilitating improved patient outcomes.

References

Barbarowicz, P., Nelson, M., DeBusk, M.R. and Haskell, W. (1980) A comparison of in-hospital education approaches for coronary bypass patients. *Heart and Lung* 9: 127–133.

Casey, E., O'Connell, J. and Price, J. (1984) Perceptions of educational needs of patients after myocardial infarction. *Patient Education and Counselling* 6(2): 77–82.

Chan, V. (1990) Content areas for cardiac teaching: patients' perceptions of the importance of teaching content after myocardial infarction. *Journal of Advanced Nursing* 15: 1139–1145.

Close, A. (1988) Nurses need to become better patient educators. *Nurse Education Today* 7: 289–291.

Conn, V.S., Taylor, S.G. and Wiman, P. (1991) Anxiety, depression, quality of life and self-care among survivors of myocardial infarction. *Issues in Mental Health Nursing* 12: 321–331.

Doak, C.C., Doak, L.G. and Root, J.H. (1985) *Teaching Patients With Low Literacy Skill.* Philadelphia: J.B. Lippincott.

Dobbels, F., De Guest, S., Vanhees, L., Katelijne, K., Schepens, K., Fagard, R. and Vanhaecke, J. (2002) Depression and the heart: a systematic overview of definition, measurement, consequences and treatment of depression in cardiovascular disease. *European Journal of Cardiovascular Nursing* 1(1): 45–55.

Duyree, R. (1992) The efficacy of in-patient education after MI. *Heart and Lung* 21(3): 217–225.

Fletcher, V. (1987) An individualised teaching programme following primary uncomplicated myocardial infarction. *Journal of Advanced Nursing* 12: 195–200.

Gambling, T. (2003) A qualitative study into the informational needs of coronary heart disease patients. *International Journal of Health Promotion and Education*, 41(3): 68–76.

Gerard, P. and Peterson, L. (1984) Learning needs of cardiac patients. *Cardiovascular Nursing* 20: 7–11.

Gessner, B.A. (1989) Adult education the cornerstone of patient teaching. *Nursing Clinics of North America* 24(3): 589–595.

Hijeck, W.T. (1984) The health belief model and cardiac rehabilitation. *Nursing Clinics of North America* 19(3): 449–456.

Howard, S. (1993) Accreditation of prior learning. Andragogy in action or a 'cut price' approach to education. *Journal of Advanced Nursing* 18: 1817–1824.

Jans, N.H. and Becker, M.H. (1984) The health belief model: A decade later. *Health Education Quarterly* 11, 1–7.

Jaarsma, T. (1999) Developing a supportive-educative program for patients with advanced heart failure within Orem's General Theory of Nursing. In: Jaarsma, T. *Heart Failure: Nurses Care Effects of Education and Support by a Nurse on Self-Care, Resource Utilization and Quality of Life of Patients with Heart Failure.* Maastricht: Dadtwyse Maastricht. (PhD Thesis).

Jaarsma, T., Kastermans, M., Dassen, T. and Philipsen, H. (1995) Problems of cardiac patients in early recovery. *Journal of Advanced Nursing* 21: 21–27.

James, P. and Dickoff, J. (1982) Toward a cultivated but decisive pluralism for nursing. In: McGee, M. (ed) *Theoretical Pluralism Nursing Science.* Ottowa: Ottowa University Press.

Jarvis, P. (1985) *The Sociology of Adults and Continuing Education.* Worcester: Routledge.

Johnston, J.L. and Morse, J.M. (1990) Regaining control: the process of adjustment after myocardial infarction. *Heart and Lung* 19(2): 126 –135.

Jowett, N.I. and Thompson, D.R. (2000) *Comprehensive Coronary Care*, 2nd edn. London: Baillière Tindall.

Karlik, B.A. and Yarcheski, A. (1987) Learning needs of cardiac patients: a partial replication study. *Heart and Lung* 16(5): 544–551.

Kettuen, S., Solovieva, S., Laamanen, R. and Santavirta, N. (1999) Myocardial infarction, spouses' reactions and their need for support. *Journal of Advanced Nursing* 30(2): 479–488.

Knowles, M.S. (1989) *The Adult Learner: A Neglected Species*, 3rd edn. Houston: Gulf Publishing Company.

Ladwig, K.H., Roll, G., Breithardt, G., Budde, T. and Borggrefe, M. (1994) Post infarction depression and incomplete recovery six months after acute myocardial infarction. *Lancet* 343: 20–23.

Lewin, B., Rolerston, I.M., Irving, J.B. and Campbell, M. (1992) A self-help post myocardial infarction rehabilitation package – the heart manual: effects on psychological adjustment, hospitalization and GP consultation. *Lancet* 339: 1036–1040.

Luker, K. and Caress, A. (1989) Rethinking patient education. *Journal of Advanced Nursing* 14: 711–718.

Mason-Attwood, H. and Ellis, J. (1971) The concept of need: an analysis for adult education. *Adult Leadership* 19: 210–212.

Merriam, S.B. (1987) Adult learning and theory building: a review. *Adult Education Quarterly* 37: 187–198.

Milazzo, A. (1980) A study of the difference in health knowledge gained through formal and informal teaching. *Heart and Lung* 9(6): 1079–1982.

Mirka, T. (1994) Meeting the learning needs of post myocardial infarction patients. *Nurse Education Today* 14: 448–456.

Moser, D. and Dracup, K. (1995) Psychosocial recovery from a cardiac event: the influence of perceived control. *Heart and Lung* 24(4): 273–280.

Moynihan, M. (1984) Assessing the educational needs of post-myocardial infarction patients. *Nursing Clinics of North America* 19(3): 441–447.

Mullen, P.D., Maims, D.A. and Velez, R.V. (1992) A meta analysis of controlled trials of cardiac patient education. *Patient Education and Counseling* 19: 143–162.

Naidoo, J. and Wills, J. (1994) *Health Promotion Foundations for Practice*. London: Ballière Tindall.

Noble, C. (1991) Are nurses good patient educators. *Journal of Advanced Nursing*. 16: 1185–1189.

Nolan, M. and Nolan, J. (1998) Rehabilitation: scope for improvement in practice. *British Journal of Nursing* 7(9): 522–526.

Oberst, M. (1989) Perspectives on research in patient teaching. *Nursing Clinics of North America* 24: 621–628.

Orem, D.E. (2001) *Nursing: Concepts of Practice*, 6th edn. London: Mosby.

Prochaska, J.O. and DiClemente, C.C. (1982) Transtheoretical therapy: towards a more integrative model of change. *Psychotherapy: Theory, Research and Practice*, 19: 276–288.

Prochaska, J.O. and DiClemente, C.C. (1984) *Transtheoretical Approach. Crossing Boundaries of Therapy*. Homewood, IL: Dow-Jones-Irwin.

Rosenstock, I.M. (1974a) The historical origins of the health belief model. In: Becker, M.H. (ed) *The Health Belief Model and Personal Health Behavior*. New Jersey: Charles B. Slack.

Rosenstock, I.M. (1974b) The health belief model and illness behavior. In: Becker, M.H. (ed) *The Health Belief Model and Personal Health Behavior*. New Jersey: Charles B. Slack.

Russell, G. (1999) *Essential Psychology for Nurses and Other Health Professionals*, London: Routledge.

Ruzicki, D. (1989) Realistically meeting the educational needs of hospitalized acute and short stay patients. *Nursing Clinics of North America*, 24: 629–636.

Scaffa, M.E. (1998) Development of a comprehensive theory in health education. *Journal of Health Education* 29(3): 179–185.

Scalzi, C., Burke, L. and Greenland, S. (1980) Evaluation of an in-patient educational program for coronary patients and families. *Heart and Lung* 9: 846–853.

Scott, J.T. and Thompson, D.R. (2003) Assessing the information needs of post-myocardial infarction patients: a systematic review. *Patient Education and Counseling*, June: 167–177.

Shea, E.J., Bogdan, D.F., Freeman, R.B. and Schreiner, G.E. (1985) Haemodialysis for chronic renal failure IV: psychological considerations. *Annals of Internal Medicine* 62(3): 558–563.

Sivarajan, E., Newton, K., Almes, M., Kempf, T.M., Mansfield, L.W. and Bruce, R.A. (1983) Limited effects of in-patient teaching and counseling after myocardial infarction: a controlled study. *Heart and Lung* 12: 65–73.

Smith, C.E. (1989) Overview of patient education. Opportunities and challenges for the twenty-first century. *Nursing Clinics of North America* 24(3): 583–587.

Stern, M.J., Pascale, L. and Ackermann, A. (1977) Life adjustment post myocardial infarction. *Archives of Internal Medicine* 137: 1680–1685.

Thompson, D.R. (1989) A randomized control trial of in-hospital nursing support for first time myocardial infarction patients and their partners: effects on anxiety and depression. *Journal of Advanced Nursing*, 14: 291–297.

Thompson, D.R., Ersser, S.J. and Webster, R. (1995) The experiences of patients and their partners 1 month after a heart attack. *Journal of Advanced Nursing* 22: 707–714.

Timmins, F. and Kaliszer, M. (2003) Information needs of myocardial infarction patients. *European Journal of Cardiovascular Nursing* 2: 57–65.

Turton, J. (1998) Importance of information following myocardial infarction study of the perceived information needs of patients and their spouse/partner compared with perceptions of nursing staff. *Journal of Advanced Nursing* 27: 770–778.

Webster, R.A., Thompson, D.R. and Mayou, R.A. (2002) The experiences and needs of Gujarti Hindu patients and partners in the first month after a myocardial infarction. *European Journal of Cardiovascular Nursing* 1(1): 69–76.

Whitaker, L.M. (2000) Sexual healing: caring for patients recovering from myocardial infarction. In: Cruikshank, J.P., Bradbury, M. and Ashurt, S. (eds) *Aspects of Cardiovascular Nursing*. London: Mark Allen Publishing Group.

Wiklund, I., Sanne, H., Vedin, A. and Wilhelmson, C. (1984) Psychosocial outcome one year after a first myocardial infarction *Journal of Psychosomatic Research* 28: 309–321.

Wingate, S. (1990) Post MI patients' perception of their learning needs. *Dimensions of Critical Care Nursing* 2(2): 112–118.

Zion, A.B. and Aiman, J. (1989) Level of reading difficulty in American College of Obstetrics and Gynaecology patient education pamphlets. *Obstetrics and Gynaecology* 74(6): 955–960.

Chapter 6

Research utilisation in coronary care

<table>
<tr><td>Key points</td></tr>
<tr><td>

- It is incumbent on all nurses to provide interventions that are research-based.
- Organisational barriers exist to the utilisation of research by nurses such as lack of authority and lack of time.
- Research utilisation is an innovation that requires a thoughtful systematic approach to ensure success.
- Research-based practice innovations require nurses to become change agents.
- Research-based practice innovations need to be monitored to ensure success.

</td></tr>
</table>

Introduction

It is widely recognised and accepted that nursing practice must be research based. Internationally, the use of research in nursing is regarded as a necessary step in an age of continued rapid technological development and quality care. Increasingly, practitioners are called upon to justify their practice, and ensure that it is based on sound evidence. What constitutes evidence attracts debate within the nursing domain, however, research is accepted to be one source of evidence that is essential for many aspects of nursing care. In Chapter 5, research regarding cardiac patients information needs was suggested to inform practice.

Research-based practice

Research-based nursing practice has been high on the agendas of international policy makers for a number of years. Successive UK Department of Health reports have advocated the need for research-based nursing. *Research for Health* (Department of Health 1991, 1993) was a milestone document that ensured research and development became an integral part of healthcare in the UK. In the USA, research in nursing has been conducted since the 1920s. In 1985 the National Center for Nursing Research (NCNR) was established to support clinical nursing research and dissemination of findings; in 1993, this became known as the National Institute of Nursing Research (NINR). This agency remains very active today and is a major influence on the continued growth of nursing research through the prioritising of the research agenda, provision of funds and implementation initiatives.

In order for nurses to use research in practice, the profession of nursing needs to be research active. The level of research activity varies between countries. Very often research activity is associated with the acquisition of primary and higher degrees and within a country may be correlated with the academic level of the practitioners within. Treacy and Hyde (1999) for example, attributed the dearth of nursing research in Ireland to the small numbers of nurses educated to doctorate level at that time. The linking of research activity to academic achievement also explains patterns and trends in research. In the past it was those nurses who taught other nurses who attained higher degrees. As a result their studies focused towards education, for example the initial nursing research in the USA. This gradually progressed to management issues, as more managers took additional studies and only later did patient issues take centre stage as increasing numbers of practising nurses started to conduct research as part of higher studies. Indeed, in Sweden, Kajermo et al. (1998) found that nurses reported lack of academic tradition as a barrier to research utilisation. Similar patterns emerge in other countries.

Research activity, of course, is not confined to only those pursuing studies, however, given the level of knowledge required and the financial implications of carrying out research, ward-based nurses have been less inclined to spontaneously conduct research. This situation has changed in recent decades with the recognition in many countries of the need to support research development with funding. The availability of funding either nationally or locally from government led or other initiatives has contributed to the advancement of practice in this particular area.

Doing research is only one component of research-based practice. While research needs to be carried out by only *some* nurses, it needs to be practised by *all*. This requires that research is communicated to nurses in an effective manner. The process has inherent difficulties. First, although a main source of communication is nursing journals, many researchers may not actually publish their findings, and therefore their word is not heard. In addition, even if the work is published practising nurses may not have access to the journal, or may not be in the habit of reading journals, so the message does not get across. Other issues with communication and dissemination arise when target groups, i.e. nurses, experience difficulty reading research results as the language used is often complex or the statistics are not easily understood.

For research-based practice to become a reality it needs to proceed through four distinct phases:

- research
- communication of the research
- reading and understanding the research
- research utilisation.

The final phase, research utilisation, is probably the most complex. Although some authors (Jacobson 2000) have called upon individual nurses to challenge current practice and integrate research, research findings suggest that many barriers exist within organisations that prevent nurses doing this. In addition, the process of utilisation requires a thoughtful systematic process that is adopted by an organisation rather than an individual. Using research in practice is regarded as an innovation.

For an innovation to be successfully implemented a good understanding of innovation theory is required.

A nurse, working in a coronary care unit (CCU) or other organisation, who recognises the need for changes to enable research-based practice, often does not have the authority to bring about the necessary change. Hunt identified this barrier in 1981, and studies on this topic suggest that this is still a mitigating factor. However, if nurses find it difficult to use research or recognise the need for additional research-based practice, they can alert management to the need for change by acting as a *change agent* and this is a very important function. Rogers (1996), who studied innovation theory extensively, suggests that the change agent has a crucial role in the success of innovations, and although Rogers' framework for innovation has been used widely in nursing to examine barriers to innovations and actually implement innovation, the role of the change agent in this process has received little attention.

Although barriers exist to nurses' use of research in practice, the literature on the topic indicates that nurses are favourably disposed towards research (McSherry 1997, Björkström and Hamrin 2001) and believe that nursing practice should be research based (Parahoo 2000). However, reported research-based practices are inconsistent. In a study reported in 1998, Parahoo revealed that most of the sample agreed that research was relevant and valuable to nursing; the majority (69%) agreed that nursing should become a research-based profession. However, only 34% of respondents indicated that nurses use research in practice. Rodgers (2000a) revealed that respondents' research-based practices ranging from 78% having never used a particular practice to 85% using it in one area. One of the nurse groups in Parahoo et al.'s (2000) study revealed that over 80% of the sample reported research use at least some of the time. However, when asked whether they had actually implemented findings of research in the past 2 years, 67% of the group had not. Lacey (1994) revealed that over half their group used research-based wound care intervention and Kyei (1993) reported a 72% level of research-based practice.

The reasons why nurses do not use research have been examined extensively from an international perspective and constraints within organisations such as lack of managerial support and time constraints predominate (McSherry 1997, Kajermo et al. 1998, Parahoo 2000, Retas 2000). Seven of the top 10 barriers in Parahoo's (2000) study were related to barriers within the practice setting including lack of funding, staff shortages, lack of support from managers and from colleagues. Interestingly, these latter items were also reported as items that facilitate research utilisation. Organisational and cultural barriers also emerged as a theme in McCaughan et al. (2002) interviews with nurses and in Hicks (1996) study.

For the nurse, this raises ethical, moral and professional issues. Long (2002: xvi) suggested that 'every practitioner has a responsibility to ensure that his or her practice is informed by best evidence. This evidence base includes high quality and appropriate research. There is thus a moral imperative on the practitioner to keep up to date with research'. McSherry et al. (2002) suggest that the main reason for evidence-informed nursing is to ensure the highest possible level of care, through allowing nurses to be accountable for their actions. The ultimate aim, they suggest is 'defensible practice'.

Clearly, nurses have a responsibility to ensure that the care they give is based upon reliable and valid research. Although numerous obstacles exist for nurses in this endeavour, it is essential that nurses begin to reflect on the implications of these barriers and begins to explore ways of highlighting the obstacles to employers and managers and develop means of overcoming them. By becoming change agents within practice, nurses can pave the way for research-based practice. Nurses who hold management positions within units and organisations have a particular responsibility to become change agents in this regard.

Hardiman (1998) outlined from personal experience the pivotal role that a ward manager can play in the use and dissemination of research. Hardiman (1998), now a hospital director, advocates that this research-based practice is a crucial factor in the delivery of quality care. She stated that it is essential for ward managers to have clinical expertise, research awareness training, and awareness to promote research-based practice. She suggested that a component of the ward manager's role in relation to research is the development of research awareness skills, the development of formal links with nurse educators and practice development and the facilitation and support of in-service education for nurses. At a micro level the ward manager's role in fostering research-based practice involves taking responsibility for getting research evidence into practice, making time for research, developing a culture where practice is reflected on and in an environment that challenges practice.

This aspiration, unfortunately, is not always reflected in practice. In 1981, Hunt a seminal writer on this topic, suggested that nursing was 'very traditional, very ritualistic and very hierarchical' and that 'those with authority to effect change do not want to, and those who want to ... do not have the requisite authority'. She pointed out that nurses often did not use research findings because they did not know about them, they did not understand them, they did not believe them, they did not know how to apply them and they were not allowed to use them. Although this piece is now dated, there is evidence to suggest tradition and ritual still exist within aspects of nursing practice, and the barriers that she outlined to research-based practice are still prevalent. Parahoo et al. (2000) revealed reasons for *never* using research, which echo Hunt's (1981) early thoughts on the topic, and included 'lack of time' and 'no supportive culture'. This finding is supported in several other studies (Funk et al. 1991a, McSherry 1997, Walsh 1997a, 1997c, Kajermo et al. 1998, Parahoo 2000, Retas 2000, Rodgers 2000a).

One US author, Jacobson (2000), suggested that much of today's nursing practice remains entrenched in ritual and tradition, which she terms 'folklore-based nursing'. She describes a ritual as 'a formal and customarily repeated act or series of acts'. Rituals include routinely measuring intake and output and vital signs and providing verbal shift report on each patient. Tradition, on the other hand is 'the handing down of information, beliefs, and customs by word of mouth'. She suggested that ritual and tradition are 'poor substitutes for research-based nursing practice'. Strange (2001) concluded that rituals persist because they serve 'emotional and social functions' within nursing practice.

The extent of research-based practice within CCUs has not been systematically studied. However, there is some evidence to suggest that ritual and tradition still prevail in some areas. In a study by Riegel et al. (1996), 882 intensive care unit nurses were surveyed to examine the use of traditions known as 'coronary precautions', which have no basis in research evidence to support their use. Reported traditional practices included offering bedpans (34%), avoiding iced beverages (28%), avoiding vigorous back rubs (16%) and avoiding hot beverages (9%). Reigel et al. noted that complete bed baths were offered by 20% of nurses to stable, pain-free patients. However, patient care decisions were governed mainly by unit policies with few nurses expressing freedom in decision making (15%).

Jacobson (2000) suggests that the best way to 'abandon folklore-based practice' and ensure that research is used in nursing practice is to encourage individual nurses to use research. Jacobson (2000) was confident that it was the individuals, rather than the healthcare organisations who were responsible for the failure to use research in practice. Jacobson (2000) suggested that nurses often blamed lack of finance and support as reasons for failure to implement research findings, however, she highlighted the fact that 'nursing's leaders' present a different rationale for this. Jacobson (2000) stated that Fay Bower, a former president of Sigma Theta Tau, 'blamed nurses' attitudes and values, not access or ability, for under utilization of research'. Jacobson (2000) called on individual nurses to take it upon them to investigate areas of practice to examine whether they are underpinned by research. She called this approach 'Power of One model of Research-Based Practice'.

These calls for an individualistic approach may be somewhat oversimplifying the process required to ensure that nursing practice is research based. While it remains an individual nurse's responsibility to ensure that his or her practice is research based, many identified barriers exist within the clinical setting, and research utilisation is regarded by many not as an individual but an organisational process (Brett 1987, Crane 1995, Kitson et al. 1996). The utilisation of research in practice has been described as an innovation that requires a systematic collegial approach towards application. Long (2002) supports this point, suggesting that this obligation is not solely the practitioner's, this requirement must extend to the clinical manager for a service, not least to their accountability for delivering a quality service.

> The organisation, down to the ward or smallest base unit, needs to provide supportive and enabling structures and processes to facilitate evidence-based practice. Thus, there needs to be access to libraries (with on-line searching facilities), dedicated/protected time to locate, read and appraise evidence (it is not reasonable to expect this to be done outside of work time) and, perhaps most challenging, empowerment in the workplace to implement (agreed) changes in practice.
>
> Long (2002: xvi)

Barriers to research utilisation in nursing

Organisations take time to adopt innovations or new practices and involve a series of processes: progression, adaptation and facilitation (Rogers 1996). 'Diffusion of innovations' is a term used to describe models that support change and development within organisations. Diffusion of innovation theory has become synonymous with both the utilisation and study of adopting research-based practice in nursing. Rogers (1962, 1971, 1983, 1996) has described one method of *diffusion of innovations*, which has frequently been used to study the nature and prevalence of obstacles (barriers) to research-based practice as an innovation in nursing practice.

The innovation process itself occurs in five stages: agenda setting; (perceived need for change); matching; redefining/restructuring and clarifying/routinising. Rogers

(1996) suggested certain variables affect the rate of adoption of innovations: the perceived attributes of the innovations; the type of innovation; the communication channels; the nature of the social systems and the extent of the change agents' promotion efforts.

In order to more fully understand the factors that affect the rate of adoption of research-based practice within nursing situations, the diffusion of innovations framework described by Rogers (1962, 1971, 1983, 1996) was utilised by Funk et al. (1991b). In particular, aspects of the perceived attributes of innovations were formalised into survey format to describe nurses' attitudes to attributes and type of innovation, communication channels and the nature of the social systems. Characteristics of the adopter were also incorporated into the instrument, which Rogers (1962, 1971, 1983, 1996) described as factors that when present in an individual, predicted their likelihood of adopting the innovation. The survey initially involved distribution of a 29-item questionnaire to a sample of 1989 US nurses. The data were subjected to factor analysis to group responses into clusters. Four main factors emerged (28 items): the characteristics of the organisation, the characteristics of the adopter, the characteristics of the communication and the characteristics of the research. The instrument was found to be reliable and was then used to collect data on barriers in many subsequent studies (Dunn et al. 1997, Walsh 1997a, 1997b, 1997c, Kajermo et al. 1998, 2000, Parahoo 2000, Retas, 2000, McCleary and Brown 2003). While the majority of studies were based in the UK, Kajermo's studies were carried out in Sweden, Retas' in Australia and the most recent study, McCleary and Brown (2003), was based in Canada. These studies revealed that the characteristics of the organisation often presented the greatest barrier to the utilisation of research. Walsh (1997b) describes this as a paradox, in other words: practice is perceived as the biggest obstacle to change in practice. The characteristics of the organisation are subdivided into eight items such as lack of authority, time, co-operation from other staff, facilities for implementation and difficulty generalising research findings to ones own setting (Funk et al. 1991b).

In a recently published study (McCleary and Brown 2003) the barriers scale (Funk et al. 1991b) was used to examine the perceived barriers to research utilisation among 176 paediatric nurses in a Canadian setting. McCleary and Brown reported the findings in rank order and the most frequently cited barrier was lack of time to read research. Relevant literature not compiled in one place ranked second. Lack of understanding of statistical analysis ranked third, insufficient authority to change client care procedures ranked fourth and insufficient time on the job to implement new ideas ranked fifth. Lack of time also ranked first in Retas' (2000) study of barriers to research utilisation in Australia and emerged as a barrier to 84% of respondents in McSherry's (1997) study.

It is interesting to note that of the studies that examined barriers to research utilisation using the barriers scale (Funk et al. 1991b, Dunn et al. 1997, Walsh 1997a, 1997b, 1997c, Kajermo et al. 1998, 2000, Parahoo 2000, Retas 2000, McCleary and Brown 2003), no one individual item emerged consistently at the top. However, three individual subscale items were consistently ranked in the top five individual items, when responses to items were placed in rank order. These were 'nurse does not feel she/he has enough authority to change patient care procedures', 'there is insufficient time on the job to implement new ideas' and 'statistical analysis are not understandable'. It is evident from these findings that the main barriers to research-based nursing practice are inherent features of the organisation structure and process. Insufficient support from management echoes throughout the literature and is an issue that must be considered by all managers of healthcare organisations and individual units.

Nurses must be empowered, as Hardiman (1998) and Long (2002) described, at local level to read research and use it in practice. The nurse manager requires trans-formational leadership qualities to make practice research-based. They need to create a vision for staff that they themselves believe and subscribe to, and they must harness the energy of staff, especially those who are potential change agents, in order to sustain the vision (Hein 1998). They need to adequately select and utilise frameworks for diffusion of research innovations such as that of Rogers (1996). Adequate facilities, including access to journals/libraries and sufficient time are crucial to the successful implementation of research-based practice. This will encourage the reading of research and facilitate understanding. The latter may be supported by locally-based research appreciation courses. A key feature of these will be the understanding of research methods and the development of the ability to read and critically analyse research studies.

However, albeit the organisation is crucial to the utilization of research, the knowledge, skills and attitudes of individual nurses to research also play their part. Closely ranked behind the organisational barriers is the subgroup of obstacles relevant to the presentation and accessibility of research papers. 'Lack of understanding of statistics' is overall the biggest issue and can be closely associated to 'research not clear/readable'. While accessibility and the quality of published research is an issue, Kajermo et al. (1998), in a study of 236 nurses, found that library services were available but not used. It is also clear that reading and interpreting research poses difficulty for some nurses.

McCleary and Brown (2003) noticed, as in other similar studies, that a lot of nurses choose the category 'no opinion', in fact there were a lot of no responses to items, resulting in a lot of missing data. In the past this was postulated to relate to nurses' lack of knowledge, and McCleary and Brown (2003) supported this hypothesis by making comparisons within the data. They found that those who had conferred no opinion to more than half of the items also reported lower levels of understanding of research design, reading research articles in journals, using research in clinical practice and conducting a literature search.

Nurses' lack of knowledge in the area of research appears to prevail as an obstacle to research utilisation, supporting early findings (Hunt 1981). The extent to which this affects practice in this area is unclear. Certainly, nurses in many studies reported difficulty understanding statistics as a barrier to utilisation, although this could be a reflection on the studies themselves as much as nurses' knowledge. Measurement of nurses' research values, skills and awareness is incorporated into the barriers scale under the *characteristics of the nurse*. In this section, 'lack of research evaluation skills' was an important factor in many studies (Dunn et al. 1997, Walsh 1997a, 1997b, 1997c, Parahoo 2000). 'Lack of awareness' was identified by 75% of respondents as a great/moderate barrier in Funk et al.'s (1991a) original study and by 67% of nurses in Dunn et al.'s (1997) study.

Kyei (1993), in the Netherlands, revealed that 60% of nurses reported that they found journals difficult to read. The most common reason cited for failure to read these were the research terminology used and the presentation of statistics. Brown (1995) highlighted the need for the research message to be simple. He suggests that the 'research message must be encoded in language which is appropriate to the intended users ... nurse researchers might do well to consider reporting their findings in academic writing for their academic supervisors and additionally in practical language for consumption by clinical practitioners'. Research language also emerged as an issue in Björkström and Hamrin's (2001) and McCaughan et al.'s (2002) studies.

In several studies, nurses were asked about their use of research resources, frequency of reading journals and accessing libraries and interesting results found. Rodgers (2000b) conducted a survey in the UK and found that the most commonly cited resource was the library (to which 90% of the sample had access), 34% of respondents received a circulation of research summaries and 39% of respondents stated that the ward receives nursing journals.

In Björkström and Hamrin's (2001) Swedish study, half of the respondents reported never having read nursing journals. In each of eight journal categories at least 60% of respondents reported that they never read the journal, and at least 22% of respondents did not respond to questions pertaining to each journal. In reality, therefore less than 18% of respondents were known to actively read research reports at least sometimes.

Parahoo et al. (2000) in the UK found that most nurses reported that they read research studies; over 50% reported that they read at least two or three monthly. *The Nursing Times*, was cited by 64% of respondents as their main source of research information. Only 12% reported accessing the *Journal of Advanced Nursing*. McSherry (1997) revealed lack of confidence in reading research as a barrier, with only 53.4% of respondents having received formal tuition on the topic. This lack of confidence also emerged in McCaughan et al.'s (2002) study.

Accessing resources was a point emphasised by Estabrooks et al. (2003) who surveyed over 7000 nurses in Canada at two separate time points, 1996 and 1998, to ascertain their access to and use of electronic and other resources. The findings revealed that over half of the 1998 group (66.1%) had access to computers at home, representing an average increase of almost 10% from 1996. However, access to computers at work was surprisingly low at 57.8%. Email use increased from 22% to 28%, however its use for work was low.

In the 1998 survey they also asked whether nurses used the internet to look up nursing information and 16.6% reported that they did so at home, with only 5% doing this at work. Estabrooks et al. (2003) also compared nurses' use of computers to that of householders and physicians in Canada, using national survey data. This comparison revealed that nurses were less likely to use computerised resources; 78% of physicians reported using a home computer and half of them use email, and 47% of physicians reported using the internet to access bibliography databases. Less than 17% of nurses reported this type of usage. Nurses compared favourably with the public, in that 27% used the internet at home compared with only 22% use by the public. However, interestingly, the public had greater access to email at work (23%) compared with nurses (5%). Clearly nurses' use of technological resources to support research use could be improved.

This point was endorsed in Thompson et al.'s (2001a) study, which revealed that the main type of information sources available to the nurses were journal articles, local policies and files and newsletters and to a lesser extent textbooks. The nurses themselves felt that accessing information direct from individuals was most reliable. The clinical nurse specialist was a common resource. During 180 hours of observation, only two forms of text-based research information were used: local protocols and guidelines and the *British National Formulary* (BNF). However, online databases were perceived as relatively accessible, but rarely used. A significant finding of the study was that those nurses working in CCU were more likely to have a positive attitude to the use of technology to guide practice and access resources.

A further emerging theme of this study was 'blending research, technology and experience for usefulness', i.e. nurses viewed summaries of research more valuable than a single research study. Nurses valued library resources, however, library skills were found to be quite basic, with several respondents avoiding electronic resources altogether. Observational data from within one library revealed that some nurses accessed electronic resources, but this was almost exclusively linked to academic courses of study.

Research-based practice is dependent upon the reading and understanding of research and based on the above account needs urgent attention. Online resources and use of libraries with reference databases should be available to all practising nurses so that up-to-date research can be adequately accessed. Long (2002) emphasised the point that time needs to be set aside for nurses to read research and should not be expected to become a requirement of their free time. Reading research can also be facilitated by local initiatives such as journal clubs where staff read and present on topics or through the provision of in-service seminars and workshops on research topics.

Provision of knowledge to practising nurses is also an area that requires attention. Previous education in research affects nurses' ability to read and use research (Ehrenfeld and Eckerling 1991, Rodgers 2000b). Rodgers (2000b) found that nurses felt attendance at higher education made them more knowledgeable and able to seek out research and evaluate it for practice.

Future innovations

Clearly, research utilisation is a complex process that involves individuals and organisations at a variety of levels. As discussed in the previous section, several barriers exist to the use of research in practice relating to the organisation itself, including managers' support and time, the communication of research, its accessibility and relevance to nurses and factors related to the nurses themselves such as research knowledge and education. In order for research-based practice to become a reality within coronary care, systematic steps must be taken to ensure that these barriers are addressed.

Several models have been used in the USA to enhance research utilisation. These include Goode's research utilisation model (Goode et al. 1987), the Stetler model (Stetler 1994) and the Iowa model of research in practice (Titler et al. 1994). Similarities exist between these models. They are implicitly prescriptive as they indicate the steps and activities of research utilisation and promote the evaluation of research findings. Two models, in particular, have been consistently used as frames of reference for studies conducted on barriers of research utilisation: the diffusion of innovation model (Rogers 1983, 1996) and the conduct and utilisation of research in nursing (CURN) model (Horsley et al. 1983).

The diffusion of innovation model (Rogers 1996) is a clear and concise theory that describes the innovation–decision process, which acts as a useful framework for healthcare practice changes. According to Rogers (1996) diffusion is the process whereby innovation is communicated within a system. Rogers (1996) describes six phases of the process of adopting an innovation, the 'innovation-development process'. This begins with recognising that there is a need or problem; performing basic or applied research into the topic; development; commercialisation (marketing); diffusion and adoption; and the consequences. In the first phase the individual nurse (or team of nurses) recognises the need or problem (e.g. the requirement to base a particular aspect of practice upon research). The next step (research) involves eliciting the views and current practice of the staff, literature search and critical analysis of the studies found. At this stage setting up a formalised team to perform duties is useful. These duties are time-consuming and require involvement of other staff. The studies are then developed into a viable proposal for the unit or organisation, which can then be marketed by the group, and hopefully diffused and adopted. Consequences should then be measured using evaluation techniques. The group involved will pass from the point of knowledge of the innovation to confirmation of the decision to implement. This process, called as 'innovation decision process', consists of five phases: knowledge, persuasion, decision, implementation and confirmation. The selected group will actively be involved in planning and co-ordinating all five phases.

Success of the innovation may be dependent upon staff involved having the required time to devote to the project. The time consuming nature of the process was highlighted by Hunt in 1987 in response to a *Nursing Times* editorial in 1983, in which it was proclaimed that 'very few people have taken up the challenge of putting research into action'. Hunt described how nurse teachers from nine schools of nursing explored the literature to enable them to underpin their teaching and practices in the hospital with research. This process took 2 years to complete.

Similarly, Loveridge (2002) describes the inherent challenges in responding to the responsibility of all practising nurses to base practice on research. She is a busy practice development adviser (PDA) in a hospital in the UK, and ensuring that practice is based on research is a major part of her role. She describes how this does not simply mean critiquing a research study and implementing it the following day; it refers to a painstaking time-consuming process which she terms 'a fact finding mission'. It is not, she points out, just a case of locating the literature, but 'assuring the reliability and validity of the resulting evidence'. After this, there is the process of proposing the findings to the 'multi-disciplinary team, thereby ensuring consensus and acceptance for any proposed change in practice'.

In some case studies clinicians have outlined the steps they have taken to implement research-based practice in one particular area of practice (Lundin and Burke 1998, Lefler 2002, Loveridge 2002) using a variety of frameworks to guide the process.

In 1998, Lundin and Burke reported on a local US innovation in 1995 using the

Iowa model. The staff had questioned the length of required bed rest at the hospital for patients following cardiac angiography. A research utilisation project team was set up to identify whether it was safe to ambulate these patients at an earlier stage than current practice dictated. The team found 14 studies through computerised database searching. The resultant outcome was reduction in bed rest to 4 hours with an estimated cost saving of U$33,000 a year.

Similarly, Lefler (2002) used the Stetler model to explore reasons why women delay seeking treatment for myocardial infarction. In Lefler's (2002) review of the research on the topic, the six reports used indicated three main reasons for the delay. These were clinical factors, and socio-demographic and psychological factors. Practice innovations included targeting at-risk groups such as elderly women for individual education. In addition, generalised information was provided to groups of women about myocardial infarction, and symptoms, including altered symptoms, that may occur in women.

Loveridge (2002) used the process of evidence-based practice adapted from McSherry and Haddock (1999) to examine the delay in patients receiving thrombolysis in hospital emergency departments. Loveridge (2002) used computerised databases to search for the relevant literature and found 29 articles. The findings supported the need for thrombolysis to be delivered promptly. It also highlighted reasons for delays in treatment such as the decision-making process between doctors. Nurse-led thrombolysis was recommended to reduce delays in treatment.

These three innovations (Lundin and Burke 1998, Lefler 2002, Loveridge 2002) highlighted that the use of a systematic process for the adoption of research-based nursing interventions is crucial to success. They also demonstrated the success and satisfaction achieved through systematically exploring the research base that informed their practice. These researchers are not advising practitioners to adopt clinical interventions, but rather aimed to emphasise the benefits to be had from using a systematic process to adopting research-based coronary care nursing practice. It is also important to recognise that these ventures were all team efforts, and involved a multi-disciplinary, rather than an individual approach; although the initial idea was often prompted by one person, highlighting the importance of a change agent within an organisation.

These frameworks provide structure, to what could otherwise be an ad hoc process. There is little empirical work that confirms the benefit of one framework over another, and they contain broadly similar stages that take the clinician from the point of the problem or question in/of practice, through researching the topic, to adopting the innovation. Rogers' (1996) diffusion of innovations theory has a lot to contribute to this area, as it provides for a greater understanding of not only the process itself but also of the complex interplay of inter-related factors, such as items which affect the speed of adoption of innovation and the importance of communication within systems. The fact that so many empirical studies have used this framework to identify barriers to research utilisation, means that there is significant theoretical development within this area and this should be further advanced. One emerging item is the 'characteristics of the organisation' shown in many studies to affect the rate of adoption of research innovations. Therefore any attempt using this framework to implement research-based practice must specifically address organisational issues during the process. This awareness will contribute to innovation success. The knowledge of barriers gleaned from studies on research utilisation is likely to integrate well with use of this framework.

When implementing research innovations the group will pass from the point of knowledge of the innovation to confirmation of the decision to implement – the innovation decision process (Rogers 1996). This means that the process is more than the collection and critical analysis of studies, it also requires that the staff, including the multi-disciplinary team are informed of the results of the literature search so that they may be persuaded of its benefits to practice and proceed to implement it. This point was clearly demonstrated in Loveridge's case (2002) where collated results of studies of bed rest requirements following angiography were presented to the cardiologists, some of whom took more time to convince, but whom all ultimately proceeded to implement, confirm and stay with this change of practice.

Overcoming resistance

Rogers (1996) highlighted that the characteristics of the organisation, the communication, the adopter and the change agent's efforts all have an impact on the speed with which innovations are adopted. In general terms, consideration needs to be given to resistance to change when new practices are advocated. McSherry and Simmons (2002) identified that resistance to change is common when considering adopting research-based practice. Resistance may be due to fear, threat, perceived loss of power, or lack of knowledge (Daft and Marcic 2001). Given that research knowledge deficits exist in practice, it is not surprising that resistance occurs and this should be anticipated.

A key element in overcoming resistance is team building within the organisation (or unit) and staff involvement at all levels of the innovation. This will improve internal relationships and people's ability to cope with environmental change (Daft and Marcic 2000). Getting all staff members involved from an early stage is essential. Celebrating early successes (Hein 1998), is an example of the leadership required to develop the team (Daft and Marcic 2000). It may be a long and arduous task for the staff involved. Organising small celebrations to mark successes can therefore improve morale. Also essential to this development is seeking the staff's views and feedback through surveys. The innovation could be preceded by an analysis of the staff's attitude to research or barriers that exist in the unit/organisation.

It is often not the change itself that is resisted, but the manner in which change is managed. Regarding research-based practice as an innovation that requires careful planning and a systematic process is less likely to yield resistance. It is also important for those involved in the innovation to understand the stages of change (Lewin 1952) that individuals' progress through during this time (see Chapter 4). McSherry and Simmons (2002: 132) suggested that this understanding may 'help to reduce obstacles that may be encountered' when implementing research-based practice. This model outlines the fundamental phases to the change process: unfreezing, moving and refreezing. In the unfreezing phase, for change to occur individuals need to recognise that there is a need for change. Moving is where the team begins to explore and examine or adjusts and accepts the changes being implemented. Refreezing occurs after a period of time when the change has been accepted and the staff settle back into a functional unit. See Chapter 4 for a detailed discussion of stages of change.

This model could be used in conjunction with Rogers (1996) diffusion of innovations framework. The change agent, considered crucial to the innovation in Rogers' (1996) work, also has a major role in the unfreezing stage (Lewin 1952). This individual, having highlighted the need for change and taken/initiated appropriate action, then encourages and supports the staff in the initial destabilising which may occur during the unfreezing period. Rogers (1996) also described how the level of innovativeness within individuals forms a continuum of five adopter categories (innovators, early adopters, early majority, late majority and laggards) indicating that people unfreeze at different intervals and which the change agent recognises, analyses and supports. Rogers (1996) suggested that a change agent can have a positive influence on innovation-decisions and that the extent of a change agent's promotion efforts influences the rate of adoption. The change agent has a powerful role in innovation developments, recognising the need for change, establishing an information-exchange relationship, diagnosing the problem, creating intent to change, translating intent to action, stabilising adoption and preventing discontinuance and achieving a terminal relationship. They have a key role in initiating and sustaining the innovation including prevention of resistance.

A simple four-stage model: assess, plan, implement and evaluate, underpins the theoretical frameworks that exist in this area. The framework given in Table 6.1 is based on this model and can be used by nursing staff, practice developers or managers to initiate research utilisation (Pallen and Timmins 2002). This framework may support individuals, managers, departments and organisations towards developing a structured approach to research utilisation. A pivotal component of this framework is the evaluation component. Very frequently, the reporting of innovations in the literature neglects to evaluate the impact of the change which is crucial, not only to ensure optimum patient care and quality care but also to adapt innovations as required, and monitor effectiveness. Brereton (2002: 16) suggests that when applying evidence to practice the final step is evaluation. She suggests that the effect of the intervention and change should be monitored as 'without evaluation the process of evidence-informed practice is at risk of exchanging old rituals for new and the effectiveness of the nursing intervention remains unknown and questionable'.

Summary and conclusions

It is the responsibility of every practising nurse in coronary care to base healthcare interventions upon valid and reliable evidence. Research forms an essential component of the evidence required for good practice, and research utilisation has received much attention in the literature. Research utilisation by nurses is described as an innovation that requires careful planning, organisation and collaboration at an organisational level. The individual nurse, recognising the need for change may act as a change agent. This pivotal role, initiates the need to question practice, and convinces others of the need for change. Case studies of innovations reveal, that while research-based practice is a time-consuming venture, it can have important benefits for practice, such as replacing outdated practices, improving the service to patients and cost savings.

Table 6.1 Suggested framework for research utilisation

	The clinician	The organisation/setting	Research	Communication
Assess	Attitudes to research Prior knowledge levels Barriers to research	Attitudes to research Levels of funding available Levels of staffing Study day allocation for staff Level of in-service education in this area Library facilities IT facilities Level of support from other disciplines Level of time devoted to research endeavour	Accessibility to search databases Local pathways for obtaining publications Level of published and unpublished research in the specific area Availability of systematic reviews in the area Relative availability of research Time required to collect information Quality of research obtained	Ease of understanding of available research Possibility of accessing original researchers to provide sessions that may ease understanding
Plan	Identify change agent Assign key person to provide leadership in this area Methods of promoting positive response to research/preventing resistance Education sessions to increase research knowledge Regular information sessions Survey of attitudes, barriers and knowledge levels Literature search	Assign key person to deal specifically with the organisation Methods of promoting positive response to research Regular information sessions Methods of securing funding and releasing staff for projects Increase in information support (library/IT) Inform and involve other disciplines in the project	Accessibility to search databases Search of research in clearly defined area Consistent pathways for obtaining information Realistic time-frame for collection based on the topic Select team/individual to carry this task out Critical review of studies obtained Development of standard/policy/practice from information obtained	Designate key person to support those involved in reviewing the studies Translation of studies that are difficult to understand Information sessions by seasoned researchers on the topic for all staff Information sessions with regard to the progress and outcome of the review Use of newly developed standard/policy/practice
Implement	Education sessions Assign key person Regular information sessions	Assign key person Regular information sessions Funding applications Plans for releasing staff from duty Secure additional library/IT facilities	Secure all necessary reviews and studies Critical review of studies obtained	Support for those involved in reviewing the studies Information sessions
Evaluate	Attitudes to research at end of project Knowledge levels at end of project	Attitudes to research at end of project Level of success with release of staff Level of success with funding application Level of increase in library/IT facilities	Extent to which plan was realised Quality and quantity of studies in the area Audit of standard/policy/practice put in place	Level of success in adoption of newly developed standard/policy/practice Views of the multi-disciplinary team with regard to the innovation Staff satisfaction with the venture and outcome

Adapted from: Pallen, N. and Timmins, F. (2002) Research-based practice: myth or reality? A review of the barriers affecting research utilisation in practice. *Nurse Education in Practice* 2: 99–108. With permission from Elsevier.

Research indicates that tradition and ritual still exist in nursing and this needs to be addressed. It is widely acknowledged that nurses have a positive attitude towards research, and agree with national and international calls for nursing to become research based, however, organisational constraints such as lack of time and power negate against the use of research in practice. Ward managers are in a key position to initiate change. Change agents, ward managers and other nurses can work together to challenge the research base that informs their practice. By developing an understanding of the processes involved in diffusing innovations (Rogers 1996) research-based practice may be attempted in a logical, systematic way, taking into consideration the multitude of items within organisations that affect innovation. Healthcare providers must give consideration to resources available. Library and information technology facilities are crucial to this process. Time is also essential. Healthcare providers need to support staff endeavours to develop research-based practice by allocating the time necessary to meet these demands. Only in this way will research-based practice become a reality.

References

Björkström, M.E. and Hamrin, K.F. (2001) Swedish nurses' attitudes towards research and development within nursing. *Journal of Advanced Nursing* 34(5): 706–714.

Brereton, L. (2002) Evidence into practice. In: McSherry, R., Simmons, M. and Abbott, P. (eds) *Evidence-Informed Nursing: A Guide for Clinical Nurses*. London: Routledge Press.

Brett, J.L. (1987) Use of nursing practice research findings. *Nursing Research* 36(6): 344–349.

Brown G.D. (1995) Understanding barriers to basing nursing practice upon research: a communication model approach. *Journal of Advanced Nursing* 21(1): 154–157.

Crane, J. (1995) The future of research utilization. *Nursing Clinics of North America* 30(3): 565–577.

Daft, R.L. and Marcic, D. (2001) *Understanding Management*, 3rd edn. Fort Worth: Dryden Press.

Department of Health (1991) *Research for Health. A Research and Development Strategy for the NHS*. London: Her Majesty's Stationery Office.

Department of Health (1993) *Research for Health*. London: Her Majesty's Stationery Office.

Dunn V., Crichton N., Roe B., Seers K. and Williams K. (1997) Using research for practice: a UK experience of the Barriers Scale. *Journal of Advanced Nursing* 26(6): 1203–1210.

Estabrooks, C.A., O'Leary, K.A., Ricker, K.L., and Humphrey, C.K. (2003) The internet and access to evidence: how are nurses positioned? *Journal of Advanced Nursing* 42(1): 73–81.

Ehrenfeld M. and Eckerling S. (1991) Perceptions and attitudes of registered nurses to research: a comparison with a previous study. *Journal of Advanced Nursing* 16(2): 224–232.

Funk, S.G., Champagne, M.T., Wiese, R.A. and Tornquist E.M. (1991a) Barriers to using research findings in practice: the clinician's perspective. *Applied Nursing Research* 4(2): 90–95.

Funk, S.G., Champagne, M.T., Wiese, R.A. and Tornquist E.M. (1991b) BARRIERS: the barriers to research utilization scale. *Applied Nursing Research* 4(1): 39–45.

Goode C.J., Lovett M.K., Hayes J.E. and Butcher L.A. (1987) Use of research based knowledge in clinical practice. *Journal of Nursing Administration*, 17(12): 11–18.

Hardiman, E. (1998) Nursing research and the role of the ward sister. Paper presented at 17th Annual Research Nursing and Research Conference February, Faculty of Nursing, Royal College of Surgeons in Ireland, Dublin, February 1998.

Hein, E.C. (1998) *Contemporary Leadership Behaviour: Selected Readings*, 5th edn. Philadelphia: Lippincott.

Hicks C. (1996) A study of nurses' attitudes towards research: a factor analytic approach. *Journal of Advanced Nursing* 23(2): 373–379.

Horsley, J.A., Crane, J., Crabtree, M.K. and Wood D.J. (1983) *Using Research to Improve Nursing Practice. A Guide*. New York: Grune and Stratton.

Hunt J. (1981) Indicators for nursing practice: the use of research findings. *Journal of Advanced Nursing* 6(3): 189–194.

Jacobson, A.F. (2000) Research utilisation in nursing: the power of one. *Orthopedic Nursing* 19(6): 61–65.

Kajermo, K.N., Nordstrom, G., Krusebrant A. and Bjorvell H. (1998) Barriers to and facilitators of research utilization, as perceived by a group of registered nurses in Sweden. *Journal of Advanced Nursing* 27(4): 798–807.

Kajermo, K.N., Nordstrom, G., Krusebrant, A., and Bjorvell H. (2000) Perceptions of research utilization between health care professionals, nursing students and a reference group of nurse clinicians. *Journal of Advanced Nursing* 31(1): 99–109.

Kitson A., Ahmed L.B., Harvey G., Seers K. and Thompson D. (1996) From research to practice: one organizational model for promoting research-based practice. *Journal of Advanced Nursing* 23(3): 430–440.

Kyei, M.B. (1993) Nurses' knowledge and opinions about the nursing research process in the Netherlands. *Journal of Advanced Nursing* 18(10): 1640–1644.

Lacey E.A. (1994) Research utilization in nursing practice – a pilot study. *Journal of Advanced Nursing* 19(4): 987–995.

Lefler, L. (2002) The advanced practice nurse's role regarding women's delay in seeking treatment with myocardial infarction. *Journal of the American Academy of Nurse Practitioners* 14(10): 449–456.

Lewin, K. (1952) *Field Theory in Social Science*. London: Routledge & Kegan Paul.

Long (2002) Some challenges in doing evidence-based practice. (Forward). In: McSherry, R., Simmons, M. and Abbott, P. (eds) *Evidence-Informed Nursing: A Guide for Clinical Nurses*. London: Routledge Press.

Loveridge, N.B. (2002) Using an evidence-base approach to thrombolysis. *Emergency Nurse* 10(5): 25–32.

Lundin, L. and Burke, L. (1998) Research utilization and improvement in outcomes after diagnostic cardiac catheterisation. *Critical Care Nurse* 18(5): 30–1, 34–9.

McCaughan, D., Thompson, C., Cullum, N., Sheldon, T.A., and Thompson, D.R. (2002) Acute care nurses' perceptions of barriers to using research information in clinical decision-making. *Journal of Advanced Nursing* 39(1): 46–60.

McCleary, L. and Brown, G.T. (2003) Barriers to paediatric nurses' research utilization. *Journal of Advanced Nursing* 42(4): 364–372.

McSherry, R. (1997) What do registered nurses and midwives feel and know about research? *Journal of Advanced Nursing*, 25(5): 985–998.

McSherry, R. and Haddock, J. (1998) Evidence-based health care: its place within clinical governance. *British Journal of Nursing* 8(2): 113–117.

McSherry, R. and Simmons, M. (2002) The importance of research dissemination. In: McSherry, R., Simmons, M. and Abbott, P. (eds) *Evidence-Informed Nursing: A Guide for Clinical Nurses*. London: Routledge Press.

McSherry, R., Simmons, M. and Pearce, P. (eds) (2002) An introduction to evidence-informed nursing. In: McSherry, R., Simmons, M. and Abbott, P. (eds) *Evidence-Informed Nursing: A Guide for Clinical Nurses*. London: Routledge Press.

Pallen, N. and Timmins, F. (2002) Research-based practice: myth or reality? A review of the barriers affecting research utilisation in practice. *Nurse Education in Practice* 2: 99–108.

Parahoo, K. (1998) Research utilization and related activities of nurses in Northern Ireland. *International Journal of Nursing Studies* 35: 283–291.

Parahoo, K. (2000) Barriers to, and facilitators of research utilization among nurses in Northern Ireland. *Journal of Advanced Nursing* 31(1): 89–98.

Parahoo K., Barr O. and McCaughan E. (2000) Research utilization and attitudes towards research among learning disability nurses in Northern Ireland. *Journal of Advanced Nursing* 31(3): 607–613.

Retas, A. (2000) Barriers to using research evidence in nursing practice *Journal of Advanced Nursing* 31(3): 599–606.

Riegel, B., Tomason, T. Carlson, B. and Gocka, L. (1996) Are nurses still practicing coronary precautions? A national survey of nursing care of acute myocardial infarction patients. *American Journal of Critical Care* 5: 91–98.

Rogers, E.M. (1962, 1971, 1983, 1996) *Diffusion of Innovations*, 1st, 2nd, 3rd, 4th edns. New York: The Free Press.

Rodgers S. (2000a) A study of the utilisation of research in practice and the influence of education. *Journal of Advanced Nursing* 32(1): 182–193.

Rodgers S. (2000b) The extent of research utilisation in general medical and surgical wards. *Nurse Education Today* 20(4): 279–287.

Stetler, C.B. (1994) Refinement of the Stetler/Marran, model for application of research findings to practice. *Nursing Outlook* 42(1): 15–25.

Strange, F. (2001) The persistence of ritual in nursing practice. *Clinical Effectiveness in Nursing* 5(4): 177–183.

Titler, M.G., Kleiber, C., Steelman, V., Goode, C., Rakel, B., Barry-Walker, J., Small S. and Buckwalter, K. (1994) Infusing research into practice to promote quality care. *Nursing Research*, 43(5): 307–313.

Thompson, C., McCaughan, D., Cullum, N., Sheldon, T., Mulhall, A., and Thompson, D.R. (2001a) The accessibility of research-based knowledge for nurses in United Kingdom acute care settings? *Journal of Advanced Nursing* 36(1): 11–22.

Thompson, C., McCaughan, D., Cullum, N., Sheldon, T., Mulhall, A., and Thompson, D.R. (2001b) Research information in nurses clinical decision-making: what is useful? *Journal of Advanced Nursing* 36(3): 376–388.

Treacy, M.P. and Hyde, A. (1999) Contextualising Irish nursing research. In: Treacy M.P. and Hyde A. (eds) *Nursing Research Design and Practice*. Dublin: University College Dublin.

Walsh, M. (1997a) Barriers to research utilisation and evidence based practice in A&E nursing. *Emergency Nurse* 5(2): 24–27.

Walsh, M. (1997b) Perceptions of barriers to implementing research. *Nursing Standard* 11(19): 34–37.

Walsh, M. (1997c) How nurses perceive barriers to research implementation. *Nursing Standard* 11(29): 34–39.

Chapter 7

Nurse-led services in coronary care

Key points

- Nurse-led care is becoming increasingly popular in the multi-disciplinary treatment of heart failure.
- Where nurse-led heart failure facilities have been established, the advice and support offered to clients has resulted in fewer re-admissions.
- Where a need has been identified for a nurse-led service, consideration needs to be given to the setting up of the programme.
- There are reports in the UK and US of the success and growth of nurse-led services in other areas of cardiology such as cardiac rehabilitation, risk factor management, smoking cessation and lipid clinics.
- Key issues need to be resolved including the monitoring of the role and actions of these nurses and their level of autonomy.

Introduction

While nurses have always had a pivotal role to play in the delivery of healthcare services to cardiac patients, evidence is increasing that the co-ordination of particular aspects central to patient care by nurses is extremely effective. There is also an emerging trend for nurses not only to co-ordinate the treatment by the healthcare team, but also to initiate the first-line treatment, in line with agreed multi-disciplinary protocols. These roles are developing independently on an international basis for a variety of reasons. First, the recognition of the growing complexity of healthcare warrants the delegation of certain aspects of medical care to suitably qualified professionals such as nurses. Secondly, trends in recent years towards the provision of quality care have improved our understanding of the gaps that may exist in service provision. In many cases, nurses are not only suitably qualified but also strategically placed to implement the changes required to bring about seamless care.

Thompson (2002) suggested that nurses are 'well placed' due to a tradition of working closely with families and patients as well as within a multi-disciplinary team. This places them in an ideal position to implement nurse-led programmes. The National Audit Office (NAO) of the National Health Service (NHS) in the UK also recognised the suitability of nurses to promote quality initiatives such as reducing hospital waiting times for patients (Lipley 2001).

Current initiatives

McMurray and Stewart (1998) highlighted that gaps existed in healthcare provision for patients with chronic heart failure (CHF). '[I]t seems clear that we can do more for patients with CHF.' One of their key recommendations was improving education for this patient group, in particular, in relation to medication. This area has witnessed unparalleled emergence of nurse-led care. De Loor and Jaarsma (2002) revealed a huge expansion in provision of services in the Netherlands in the past 5 years. While few programmes existed in the early 1990s, by 1999 there were 20 and this figure doubled in the following year.

CHF is a common and debilitating condition (Gould 2002). While the mortality from coronary heart disease appears to be declining in Western countries, hospital admission for heart failure appears to be on the increase (Sharpe and Doughty 1998). McMurray and Stewart (2001) described this phenomenon as 'the increasing burden of chronic heart failure', 'the residual effects of better health-care strategies ...' (2001: 1), thus suggesting that ever advancing treatment modalities for acute cardiac conditions contribute to better survival rates and an increasing population that is susceptible to heart failure.

Of particular concern internationally are the increasing costs of treating this condition, most notably frequent hospital admissions. Blue and McMurray (2001) noted that in the UK heart failure is the most common and the most expensive cause of admission in people over 65 years of age. Cost concerns were also reported in Sweden (Cline and Iwarson 2001) and the USA (Martens 2001). The potential costs associated with this particular condition have prompted innovative and integrated approaches to treatment and contributed to the emergence of the nurse-led era.

There is an increasing momentum in the UK, Ireland, Australia and many parts of Europe to manage patients with CHF on an outpatient, nurse-led basis (Warburton 2002). This is not only to reduce the costs associated with hospitalisation, but also to improve patient outcome and quality of life through the provision of a co-ordinated specialist monitoring, support and advice service. There is growing evidence that this service, particularly where a home-based element exists, has the potential to significantly reduce the number of hospital re-admissions in this patient group, thus reducing hospital costs. In addition, it has been found to have a positive impact on the quality of life of many patients (De Loor and Jaarsma 2002).

Lasater (1996) and Blue et al. (2001) found that the nurse-led intervention for patients with CHF resulted in fewer re-admissions than usual care. Stewart et al. (1999) reported that nurse-led home-based intervention resulted in fewer events and significantly fewer re-admissions. Blue and McMurray (2001) noted a 50% reduction in re-admission for heart failure with a nurse-led service in the UK. Stewart and Horowitz (2001) concluded from their study that 'a relatively inexpensive, specialist nurse-led intervention augments the efficacy of pharmacotherapy in limiting re-admission to hospital and death in a group of patients with severe, chronic heart failure over a period of at least 6 months'. They suggested that nurse-led care in heart failure 'has the potential to significantly improve health outcomes in individuals with severe, chronic heart failure... it represents an attractive adjunct to the current management of chronic heart failure ...'.

CHF is associated with exercise intolerance, dyspnoea, breathlessness, oedema, fatigue and premature death (McMurray and Stewart 2001, Gould 2002). Although many causes exist for its onset, CHD is the most frequent contributory factor (Gould 2002). The underlying physiological cause for heart failure is most commonly left ventricular dysfunction (Gould 2002).

In practice, it has been seen that patients with CHF are frequently re-admitted to hospital due to worsening of symptoms. Where nurse-led facilities have been put in place, the advice and support offered to clients has resulted in fewer re-admissions (Stewart et al. 1999, Blue and McMurray 2001, Stewart and Horowitz 2001). Hospital-based programmes typically follow patients after discharge following an acute event (De Loor and Jaarsma, 2002). Having such access to one or more nurses, who understand the patient's condition and personal situation makes it easier for the patient to call upon the service when symptoms first start and receiving appropriate advice. Much of the work of the nurse in the service concerns supporting the pharmacological management of the patient through education and support. Programmes commonly aim to reduce the need for hospital re-admission, empower individuals to manage their treatment regimens and improve their quality of life (De Loor and Jaarsma 2002). The nurse assesses the patient's knowledge level regarding medication and its use and education is provided accordingly.

Warburton (2002) suggested that education is a vital component of nurse-led heart failure programmes. Very often the patient is not fully aware of their condition and its implications for their life. Education of patients should involve understanding and recognising signs and symptoms of deterioration of the condition, advice about changing lifestyle, monitoring of weight and reporting of symptoms.

A nurse-led service may also provide general lifestyle advice, such as balancing work and rest, monitoring fluid intake and output and moderating sodium and alcohol consumption, all of which contribute to improved symptoms. Emotional support is also provided. In De Loor and Jaarsma's (2002) study, programme approaches included home visits, follow up telephone call or clinic visit. Some hospitals used only clinic visits, others combined this with a telephone call or a home visit. Blue and McMurray (2001) suggested that success of a programme depends upon regular contact with patients to detect clinical deterioration, continued adjustment and optimisation of therapy, and educating patients and families about the symptoms of heart failure and how to recognise them and who to contact when they occur.

In many cases, when patients report worsening symptoms, nurses may liaise with a physician to organise changes to medication or may give advice medication changes depending on the local policy/national guidelines on the administration of medicines. Titration of medication, namely diuretics, has become central to adequate symptom management in the community and subsequent reduction in hospital stays. In De Loor and Jaarsma's (2002) study almost 80% of the management programmes involved adjustment of medication by nurses after consulting with the physician in charge of the patient's care. In 11% of the hospital-based programme this was done independently by nurses suggesting that nurses initiated changes in medication according to local protocol without direct medical consultation in each case. Blue and McMurray (2001) strongly supported the adjustment of medication by nurses with supporting protocol. Blue and McMurray (2001), De Loor and Jaarsma (2002) and Warburton (2002) all perceived that medication adjustment is an aspect of nurse-led care that is vital to achieve its overall aims.

Current thinking also suggests that nurse-led clinics should expand the boundaries of traditional care by exploring and evaluating the benefits of home visits which are known to improve outcomes (Weinberger et al. 1996, Stewart et al. 1999). De Loor and Jaarsma (2002) found that they were 'rarely used in the Netherlands'. Blue and McMurray (2001) were quite convinced that 'developing a nurse-led heart failure clinic in conjunction with home visiting appears to be the most satisfactory way forward'.

While there is evidence of the benefits and use of nurse-led service for patients with CHF internationally, the extent of service provision is unclear, e.g. Garbett (1996) suggested that some information on development of nurse-led care in the UK is held in databases such as the King's Fund Nursing Development programme and the NHS Centre for Reviews and Dissemination but a national register may need to be developed. DeLoor and Jaarsma (2002) found that 75% of all hospitals in the Netherlands reported involved in heart failure management at some level with just over half reporting a nurse-led programme in action. Cline and Iwarson (2001) reported that nurse-led heart failure clinics are common in Sweden, with most employing a heart failure nurse. This is due in part to a long tradition of independent working by nurses with adaptation to extended roles, partially due to shortage of physicians.

Nurses are also playing an increasing role in the management of heart failure in the USA. Martens (2001) described how the advent of Diagnostic Related Groups (DRGs) in 1983 in the USA radically changed the funding of hospital care, which affected management of patients with heart failure. Comprehensive nurse-managed out-patient heart failure programmes were developed to facilitate effective management of the patients within the community.

While the benefits of nurse-led care are widely reported patients' views on this service are less understood. Wright et al. (2001) in a qualitative study described the patients' perceptions of nurse-led secondary preventive care for established coronary heart disease. The results indicated that all patients viewed nurse-led care as acceptable and were confident about nurses' ability to conduct assessments and follow up routine issues. Patients felt that the time offered by the nurses during the assessment was an advantage and quite different to the rushed atmosphere that can occur in the general practitioner's (GP) surgery. They also suggested that the nurse functioned as patient advocate and was in a good position to contact the GP if required.

Chapple and MacDonald (1999) reported patients' perceptions of a nurse-led pilot scheme in the UK. In this situation the nurse was leading a GP practice, which employed a part-time GP and other healthcare staff. Although not reported on in sufficient methodological detail, the findings did appear to indicate that confusion existed about the role and function of the nurse within the practice, with many patients believing it to be a cheaper option decision or due to shortages of GPs. Most patients, however, spoke enthusiastically about the care that they received and some patients preferred to see the nurses, believing that they had a 'deeper insight' into the patients' problems.

Thompson (2002) contended that several issues with regard to nurse-led services need to be addressed in order to ensure the appropriate development of this innovation. One issue that arises in the literature is qualification levels of nurses, with which Thompson (2002) has particular concern, urging that uniform qualification levels be adopted internationally. Similarly, there appeared to be confusion regarding the term specialist nurse in some studies, when in fact the nurse-led service was performed by a dedicated nurse, rather than a specialist nurse per se (Newman 2002; commentary on Blue et al. 2001).

Thompson (2002) also highlighted an emerging concern at practice level that some nurse-led interventions, particularly in cardiovascular care, may be perceived as of a medical or technical nature and can cause controversy. Thompson (2002) suggested exercising caution in the development of these new roles that are often contextually developed without national or standard guidelines. This is to avoid the medical model of care re-emerging at the expense of holistic patient care, which has traditionally been the nurses' domain. It is also recommended to evaluate effectiveness of the programme and initiate improvements in the role. By organising and developing the service in a systematic, collegial way clear guidelines for practice can be agreed upon.

Setting up a nurse-led service

Where a need has been identified for a nurse-led service, consideration needs to be given to the setting up of the programme. Stewart and Blue (2001a) outlined the key components establishing nurse-led programmes for the management of CHF. They suggested that some components should be considered and incorporated at the outset of planning for the service 'to ensure that it evolves into an effective one'. Ideally, this should be done by a multi-disciplinary project team whose first task should be to recruit a suitably qualified specialist nurse who can effectively manage these patients. Stewart and Blue (2001a) suggested that the nurse should be experienced in managing heart failure, be able to work independently, display initiative and be able to engender trust from both patient and the healthcare team. They did not allude to specific qualifications although it was noted that the specialist nurse described in a previous study held post-graduate qualifications in coronary care nursing (Stewart and Horowitz 2001). This is an area where some standardisation, nationally and internationally is required.

There is considerable diversity within and between countries regarding the minimum academic qualifications required for a nurse-led position. While the competencies described above may be universally required and understood, clear guidelines for the recruitment and training of these nurses is required to ensure parity of employment conditions as well as consistency in patient care. In some areas of Europe the skills and expertise required are post-graduate diploma/certificate level, although many nurses have master's degrees. In countries, such as the USA, where advanced practice is more developed, master's degree is required. The first step in this decision is outlining the required competencies and then matching the appropriate level of study. Clearly, post-graduate study at master's and PhD levels involves research, the requirement for which has not been explicitly outlined. What is crucial in nurse-led care is availability of a nurse who can manage and co-ordinate multi-disciplinary care and communicate effectively with patients. They should have knowledge and expertise in the field of cardiac nursing and heart failure management. Stewart and Blue (2001b) suggested that other skills and knowledge could be given further consideration at the interview. These may include specific experience in managing patients with heart failure, further qualifications and/or higher nursing qualifications, experience in research or audit and advanced information technology skills. Stewart and Blue (2001b) also suggested that the nurse should have been qualified at least 5 years, with at least 2 year's recent cardiology experience. They also suggested excellent communication skills, experience working in autonomous positions, ability to work in a multi-disciplinary setting, some computing skills and a driving licence. While performing research and knowledge development in the area is desirable, it may not be essential. Health service providers need to examine what is in the best interests of the patient and the nursing profession before establishing standardised guidelines. Consensus within countries and possibly between countries is advisable.

In practical terms one nurse can only practically accommodate 200 patients discharged from one hospital per year (Stewart and Blue 2001b). An alternative model is a regional approach, employing several nurses, spanning several hospitals under the direction of a regional co-ordinator. Once the requirements of staffing and service area have been decided recruitment and training may begin. Stewart and Blue (2001b) suggested that the training programme also needs to include an update on the healthcare system, heart failure, record keeping and audit and administrative issues. This may empower the chosen nurse to lead the development of the service with the relevant members of the multi-disciplinary project team. The team members need to work together to develop criteria and guidelines to guide the service.

The next phase involves deciding which patients to include within the service. There is agreement within the literature that the service should be as inclusive as possible. De Loor and Jaarsma (2002) were disappointed to find that elderly patients in nursing homes were often excluded from services. Stewart and Blue (2001a) suggested identifying *high-risk* patients. They pointed out that while treatment is effective in all classes of patients, high-risk patients are at most risk of further hospitalisation and have been found to benefit most from interventions such as this. The selection of patients may be informed by the aims and objectives of the service and involves taking a systematic, rather than piecemeal approach to programme development.

Stewart and Blue (2001b) outlined a systematic ten-step approach to establishment of a nurse-led service (Box 7.1). Given the complexity of this intervention and variety of healthcare provision on an international level it is impossible to provide a 'prescription' for constructing a service. They suggest that their recommendations serve as a 'preliminary blueprint for establishing a formalised programme'.

The first step involves a precise description of the services, with specific aims and objectives. These emerge from discussion and debate within the project team, supported by the literature. Potential healthcare users of the service (stakeholders) may be informed of the aims and objectives of the service early on, in advance of forging formal links. One of the crucial decisions is where the nurse will actually be based. Positioning this role within the hospital or community will obviously affect the nature of service delivery and patients' perception of the service. The multi-disciplinary team may decide this.

The third step is patient selection. Stewart and Blue (2001b) suggested that this should be as inclusive as possible, however, where possible patients with 'relatively

---

Box 7.1 A ten step approach to establishment of the nurse-led service

1. Develop a precise description of the services with a list of aims and objectives
2. Establish formal links with other relevant healthcare services
3. Select the type of patient eligible for intervention
4. Establish a concise protocol for admitting patients to the service
5. Establish precise operational guidelines for the service following patient discharge
6. Establish precise operational guidelines for patient follow-up
7. Auditing the service
8. Appointing and training personnel
9. Miscellaneous considerations
10. Undertake a final review of the service before formally recruiting patients

Source: Stewart, S. and Blue, L. (2001b) Establishing a specialist nurse-led service. In: Stewart, S. and Blue, L. (eds) *Improving Outcomes in Chronic Heart Failure*. London: BMJ Books, 114–118.

---

straightforward' medical conditions should be included so that they are easily managed using the guidelines. It may be prudent, for example, to exclude those with co-existing conditions that may complicate treatment. Stewart and Blue (2001b) have provided examples of inclusion and exclusion criteria for development purposes.

One critical aspect (steps 4–6) of the project team's work is to establish precise protocols for admitting patients to the service, operational guidelines for the service following patient discharge and for patient follow-up. These need to be in place in advance of setting up the service so that the boundaries of service provision are clear. This transparency paves the way for clarity and consistency of nursing actions within the service including education, advice and referral.

Auditing the service (steps 7–9) is another important activity. Structures for audit need to be put in place in advance of commencement and may be arranged by the project team. Just prior to the recruitment of patients a final review of the service should be undertaken (step 10). The aims and objectives need to be assessed to ensure realism and accuracy. Links with other services need to be clearly defined and clarified. Protocols for identifying, recruiting patients and managing patients need to be available, precise and workable. A pilot introduction period needs to be planned for.

Similar guidelines were put forward by Kimmel (1999) describing strategies for developing and implementing a nurse-managed preventive cardiology programme in the USA. Her first step is to establish the need for the service and outline the problem. Next the key stakeholders and barriers are identified (develop strategies to overcome them) network, develop a plan, and pilot the project, using this to evaluate and make adjustments and finally implement the programme. In the final analysis, to 'improve the chances of success' one should take measures to minimise resistance to change, communicate effectively, use existing resources, expect and deal with discouragement and disappointment (Kimmel 1999).

Evaluation of nurse-led services is also important, and though not directly recommended by either Stewart and Blue or Kimmel has become an integral component of nurse-led programmes to date. Evaluation provides indication of a programme's success. The outcome indicators frequently used include measurement of hospital re-admission rates, other mortality and morbidity, and quality and satisfaction. It is recommended that these evaluation methods continue and are integrated into all nurse-led programmes as a component of on-going quality and development initiatives. Increasingly, healthcare providers are becoming concerned with outcome measurement for cost and quality reasons; it is prudent therefore to continue good practice in this area.

Escalation of nurse-led services

Nurse-led services have also emerged in other areas of cardiac nursing; it has been recognised, that due to the 'burden of cardiovascular disease', some individuals fail to receive optimum care (Thompson 2002), for example delays in receiving optimum drug therapy (thrombolysis). Thompson highlighted that nurse direction has proved useful in both cardiac rehabilitation and heart failure practice, while nurse-led and nurse-initiating interventions have been particularly successful in reducing waiting times in some areas such as thrombolysis delivery.

Prompted by delays in treatment, Loveridge (2002) proposed nurse-led thrombolysis to reduce delays in drug administration within hospital settings – 'the future may see nurse-led thrombolysis as a norm …'. Indeed nurse-led care is becoming increasingly popular in the administration of thrombolysis. Holland and Foxcroft (2000) examined the 'sensitivity and specificity of coronary care unit (CCU) nurses' ability to diagnose acute myocardial infarction (AMI) and to make an independent clinical decision about thrombolysis'. They specifically considered whether or not trained nurses could diagnose AMI and initiate treatment as effectively as medical staff and whether or not nurse-led thrombolysis was time saving (door to needle), and also examined attitudes of CCU nurses towards nurse-led thrombolysis. In the study the nurses did not make real treatment decisions but rather recorded their diagnosis and choice of treatment before the arrival of medical staff.

The nurses suggested treatment choices were compared with the actual medical decisions using retrospective analysis guided by a consultant cardiologist. The specificity of nurse-led thrombolysis related to decisions not to treat was 98% compared with 94% for doctor-led (senior house officer, SHO) thrombolysis. With regard to treatment decisions, 85% of nurses were right compared with 93% of SHOs. Nurse-led thrombolysis resulted in a shorter door-to-needle time (7 minutes compared with 15 minutes with SHO-led). The attitude survey revealed that 93% of nurses (n = 13) felt confident about diagnosing myocardial infarction using ECG, and the same proportion felt confident about decision-making with regard to thrombolysis. Although the study revealed that nurses were somewhat more cautious about treatment, it did highlight their potential to contribute to this area, particularly with regard to reducing time delays. Additional training may be required to improve nurses' decision-making skills. In addition, several nurses were involved in the nurse-led procedure in this study whereas selection, recruitment and training of a designated nurse (or nurses) to lead the system would probably result in greater accuracy due to specialist skills.

Correct positioning of the nurse in the healthcare system has been a challenge to heart failure nurses, and it appears to present the same challenge to nurses leading thrombolysis. Evidence suggests that prompt administration of thrombolysis in the hospital emergency department, rather than waiting until the patient arrives to CCU, reduces possible time delays. Irrespective of whether direct admission to CCU is possible, positioning the nurse-led system within the emergency department is likely to increase time saving through rapid assessment, detection and co-ordination of care. Gamon et al. (2002) reported on an initiative in Salford, UK, whereby, an attempt to reduce the door-to-needle time for patients, patients requiring thrombolysis were assessed and treated in the emergency department rather than being fast-tracked to the CCU, as previously practised. A nurse co-ordinator was instated to co-ordinate the delivery of thrombolysis in A&E and to ensure systems were in place to support this innovation. Part of this role involved the training of nursing and medical personnel. Over a period of 2.5 years 503 patients received thrombolysis and 48% of these were judged to have been immediately eligible on admission. The median door-to-needle time was 27 minutes and 60% received thrombolysis within 30 minutes. The delay reduced from 90 minutes (prior to initiation) to 52 minutes as a result of the project.

Rhodes (1998) in a review of the literature highlighted the 'overwhelming' evidence supporting the reduction of door-to-needle by nurse-led initiatives. Nurse-led strategies impacted upon this reduction since thrombolytic therapy was administered at the point of entry to the hospital, avoiding duplication of assessments and earlier identification of potential candidates ('importance of the nursing role within these processes has been clearly established, especially in relation to the determining suitability for thrombolytic therapy', Rhodes 1998). She suggested that because of paucity of suitable research evidence further research is required to compare its accuracy and safety with medical-led care. Future research could also identify the prevalence and nature of current nurse-led interventions.

Inconsistency in nursing qualifications is an issue in nurse-led heart failure services and nurse-led thrombolysis. Holland and Foxcroft (2000) in their study, noted a minimum required qualification of post-graduate nursing certificates in 57% of cases and in less than half there was also a minimum requirement of two years CCU experience. Inconsistency exists regarding role boundaries within services. Most of the literature refers to nurse-led services, whereby the nurse co-ordinates the care given, assesses the patient and the physician initiates treatment. *Nurse-initiated* services, however, also involve the nurse administering treatment without necessarily consulting with the physician, rather instead using agreed protocols to support the assessment and expertise. Interestingly, Rhodes (1998) did not differentiate between these services in her review. This lack of uniformity and consensus on the nurse's role in nurse-managed thrombolysis services may lead to an inconsistent understanding and interpretation of the role both within and without the profession. Thompson (2002) has called for national guidelines to direct nursing role developments; this may avoid the existing lack of role clarity.

The lack of understanding of the nature of the role may have prompted respondents in Holland and Foxcroft's (2000) study to respond negatively to the proposal of nurse-led thrombolysis. Fewer than half (43%) of the nurse respondents stated that it should be part of the nurse's role. Negative comments related to the additional responsibility without renumeration and role conflict. Many nurses felt it was the doctor's duty to lead care in this area. These negative views may be due to the perception and lack of clarity regarding the boundaries of this role. A *nurse-led* service that promptly assesses patients and co-ordinates timely effective care by the healthcare team is in the best interests of the patient as it improves quality care and potential outcomes. Direct responsibility for patient assessment and co-ordination of care may be viewed as an extension of the skills of cardiac nurses. This fact, together with the potential improvement in patient care is likely to be congruent with nurses' values. Conflict may arise with the expansion of duties to include the administration of thrombolysis (*nurse-initiated*), hitherto confined to the medical domain of practice. This echoes Thompson's (2002) concern and of clinicians and academics regarding the 'over medicalisation' of the nurse's role. Clearly, direction from national representative bodies is required to adequately ascertain the most appropriate roles within the changing health service structure to respond appropriately to patients' needs with due consideration for the needs and concerns of the profession.

The extent of nurse-led thrombolysis is also unclear. Smallwood and Chadwick (2000) pointed to the difficulty with ascertaining exactly how widespread nurse-initiated thrombolysis was in one area of the UK. Following an informal telephone survey of 24 units, two were identified as using this practice with a further nine expressing an interest in this practice.

There are reports in the UK and US literature of the success and growth of nurse-led services in other areas of cardiology such as cardiac rehabilitation (Hampshire 2001), risk factor management (Campbell et al. 1998, Kimmel 1999, McHugh et al. 2001), smoking cessation clinics (Haddock and Burrows 1997, Johnson et al. 1999) and lipid clinics (Cofer 1997, Curry 2000, Jairath 2002). Another area receiving recent attention is cardioversion. Quinn (1998) reported on an observational study of 88 patients admitted to one US hospital for elective cardioversion and concluded that nurse-led day case for elective cardioversion 'appears to offer a safe alternative to CCU admission'. He pointed out that the associated legal and professional issues have attracted debate in the literature and are on-going. Many of the team felt quite strongly that this role should be given to junior medical staff, so clearly role boundaries need to be defined. For all nurse-led innovations funding issues need to be addressed. He concluded that:

> this small observational series suggests that elective cardioversion on a general medical elective ward, undertaken or under the supervision of a suitably trained nurse is a safe, feasible alternative to CCU admission. Such an approach may improve patient care by reducing the waiting times and removing the risk of the procedure being postponed due to logistical difficulties such as emergency admissions to the booked CCU bed.
>
> Quinn (1998)

Obviously, larger prospective studies are recommended in this area. However, nurse-led systems in cardiology is a welcome innovation that is likely to have a positive impact upon patient outcome, satisfaction and quality of care. Nurse-led heart failure clinics, which have been the forerunner in this advance, have met with unparalleled success. Several studies reported reductions in hospital re-admission rates for patients as well as improvements in quality of life. Nurse-led systems have been developed for other aspects of patient care, most notably, thrombolysis delivery after myocardial infarction. The impetus for this is to reduce current treatment delays, and commitment to quality patient care renders this service potentially valuable for the future.

Other areas where nurse-led incentives have been embraced include risk factor management. This is an expanding area of benefit and relevance to all patients with CHD so there is clearly a need for this service. Further research is required on the potential benefits of this service and cost implications.

Summary and conclusions

While unequivocally positive about the emergence and continued growth of nurse-led innovations, Thompson (2002) highlighted that there are 'major issues to be resolved'. He suggested that the future direction of nurse-led services needs to consider the monitoring of the role and actions of these nurses and their level of autonomy. Suitable methods of integrating this role into present healthcare structures need to be developed. He also suggested that minimum required qualifications for a (specialist) nurse need to be clearly identified. 'Given the promising results to date, it would be disappointing if these issues remain unresolved and the potential value of this type of intervention unfulfilled' (Thompson 2002).

Evaluation of current roles may be the first step in this clarification process, a point endorsed by Thompson (2002). This process could inform future developments and allow practising clinicians to more fully understand the complexities of these services. It is important that this evaluation includes the patient's perspective on the service, which has been little addressed in the literature.

In addition to evaluation, national audits may need to be performed to assess the number and function of nurse-led systems. This could form the basis of national standardised guidelines for the development, implementation and evaluation of nurse-led services including direction of the expansion of boundaries to ensure consistency, and maintain the best interests of the profession and the patient.

The development of nurse-led services represents an unprecedented challenge to cardiac nurses. There is potential scope for nurses to make a tangible impact upon patients' quality of care and quality of life. In an age of increasing professionalism, education and accountability among nurses, this challenge has been embraced. It is essential that future service development be underpinned with clear guidelines for the parameters of practice.

References

Blue, L. and McMurray, J.J.V. (2001) A specialist nurse led, home-based, intervention in Scotland. In: Stewart, S. and Blue, L. (eds) *Improving Outcomes in Chronic Heart Failure*. London: BMJ Books.

Blue, L., McMurray, J.J.V., Davie, A.P., McDonagh, T.A. and Murdoch, D.R. (2001) Randomised controlled trial of specialist nurse intervention in heart failure. *British Medical Journal* 323: 715–718.

Campbell, N.C., Ritchie, L.D., Thain, J., Deans, H.G., Rawles, J.M. and Squair, J.L. (1998)

Secondary prevention in coronary heart disease: a randomised trial of nurse led clinics in primary care. *Heart*, 80: 447–452.

Chapple, A. and MacDonald, W. (1999) A nurse-led pilot scheme: the patients perspective. *Primary Health Care*, 9(4): 16–17.

Cline, C. and Iwarson, A. (2001) Nurse-led clinics for the management of heart failure. In: Stewart, S. and Blue, L. (eds) *Improving Outcomes in Chronic Heart Failure*. London: BMJ Books.

Cofer, L.A. (1997) Aggressive cholesterol management: role of the lipid nurse specialist. *Heart and Lung*, 26: 337–344.

Curry, J. (2000) A nurse led lipid clinic. *Journal of Community Nursing*, 14(2): 6, 8, 10.

De Loor, S. and Jaarsma, T. (2002) Nurse-managed heart failure programmes in the Netherlands. *European Journal of Cardiovascular Nursing* 1: 123–129.

Gamon, R., Driscoll, P., Cooper, A., Barnes, P. and Parr, B. (2002) Can emergency department-initiated thrombolysis supported by a thrombolysis co-ordinator reduce treatment times? *Care of the Critically Ill* 18(4): 104–106

Garbett, R. (1996) The growth of nurse-led care. *Nursing Times* 92(1): 71.

Gould, M. (2002) Chronic heart failure. In: Hatchett, R. and Thompson, D. (eds) *Cardiac Nursing: A Comprehensive Guide*. London: Churchill Livingstone.

Haddock, J. and Burrows, J. (1997) The role of the nurse in health promotion: an evaluation of a smoking cessation programme in surgical pre-admission clinics. *Journal of Advanced Nursing* 26: 1098–1110.

Hampshire, M. (2001) Exercising choice: a nurse-led rehabilitation scheme is helping patients to reduce their risk of heart disease ... community-based cardiac rehabilitation programme. *Nursing Standard* 16(9): 14–15.

Holland, E. and Foxcroft, D. (2000) Is nurse-led thrombolysis clinically safe, beneficial and acceptable? *Nursing Times Research* 5(3): 227–236.

Jairath, N. (2002) Effect of behavioral nursing intervention on long-term lipid regulation. *Outcomes Management* 6(1): 34–39.

Johnson, J.L., Budz, B., Mackay, M. and Miller, C. (1999) Evaluation of a nurse-delivered smoking cessation intervention for hospitalized patients with cardiac disease. *Heart and Lung*, 28(1): 55–64.

Kimmel, L.K. (1999) Nurse-managed preventative cardiology programs. *Journal of Care Management*, 5(5): 10–18.

Lasater, M. (1996) The effect of a nurse-managed CHF Clinic on patient readmission and length of stay. *Home Health Care Nurse* 14(5): 351–356.

Lipley, N. (2001) NAO backs nurse-led clinics to ease outpatient waiting. *Nursing Standard* 15(46): 6.

Loveridge, N.B. (2002) Using an evidence-based approach to thrombolysis. *Emergency Nurse*, 10, 25–32.

Martens, K. (2001) The increasing role of nurses in the management of heart failure in the USA. In: Stewart, S. and Blue, L. (eds) *Improving Outcomes in Chronic Heart Failure*. London: BMJ Books.

McHugh, F., Lindsey, G.M., Hanlon, P., Hutton, I., Brown, M.R., Morrison, C. and Wheatly, D.J. (2001) Nurse led shared care for patients on the waiting list for coronary artery bypass surgery: a randomised controlled trial. *Heart*, 86(3): 317–323.

McMurray, J.J.V. and Stewart, S. (1998) Nurse led multidisciplinary intervention in chronic heart failure. *Heart*, 80: 430–431.

McMurray, J.J.V. and Stewart, S. (2001) The increasing burden of chronic heart failure. In: Stewart, S. and Blue, L. (eds) *Improving Outcomes in Chronic Heart Failure*. London: BMJ Books.

Newman, M. (2002) Can specialist nurse intervention reduce mortality and morbidity in patients admitted to hospital with chronic heart failure? *Evidence Based Nursing* 5(2): 55.

Quinn, T. (1998) Early experience of nurse-led elective DC cardioversion. *Nursing in Critical Care* 3(2): 59–62.

Rhodes, M.A. (1998) What is the evidence to support nurse led thrombolysis? *Clinical Effectiveness in Nursing* 2: 69–77.

Sharpe, N. and Doughty, R. (1998) Epidemiology of heart failure and ventricular dysfunction. *The Lancet* 352: 3–7.

Smallwood, A. and Chadwick, R. (2000) Nurse-initiated thrombolysis in coronary care. *Nursing Standard* 15(2): 38–40.

Stewart, S. and Blue, L. (2001a) Key components of specialist nurse-led programmes in chronic heart failure. In: Stewart, S. and Blue, L. (eds) *Improving Outcomes in Chronic Heart Failure.* London: BMJ Books.

Stewart, S. and Blue, L. (2001b) Establishing a specialist nurse-led service. In: Stewart, S. and Blue, L. (eds) *Improving Outcomes in Chronic Heart Failure.* London: BMJ Books.

Stewart, S. and Horowitz, J.D. (2001) A specialist nurse-led, multidisciplinary, home-based intervention in Australia. In: Stewart, S. and Blue, L. (eds*) Improving Outcomes in Chronic Heart Failure.* London: BMJ Books.

Stewart, S., Marley, J.E., and Horowitz, J.D. (1999) Effects of a multidisciplinary, home-based intervention on unplanned readmissions and survival among patients with chronic congestive heart failure: a randomised controlled study. *The Lancet* 354: 1077–1083.

Thompson, D. (2002) Nurse-directed services: how can they be made more effective? *European Journal of Cardiovascular Nursing* 1: 7–10.

Warburton, P. (2002) Reducing hospital readmissions for people with heart failure *Professional Nurse* 17(12): 738–740.

Weinberger, M., Oddone, E.Z., and Henderson, W.G. (1996) Does increased access to primary care reduce hospital readmissions? *New England Journal of Medicine* 334: 1190–1195.

Wright, F.L., Wiles, R.A., and Moher, M. (2001) Patients' and practice nurses' perceptions of secondary preventative care for established ischaemic heart disease: a qualitative study *Journal of Clinical Nursing* 10: 180–188.

Index